Gastrointestinal Surgery Series
MINIMAL INVASIVE HEPATOBILIARY AND PANCREAS SURGERY

Gastrointestinal Surgery Series

MINIMAL INVASIVE HEPATOBILIARY AND PANCREAS SURGERY

Editors

Dhiresh Kumar Maharjan
MRCS (Edin) FCPS
Associate Professor
Department of General and GI Surgery
Kathmandu Medical College and Teaching Hospital
Sinamangal, Kathmandu, Nepal

Prabin Bikram Thapa MS
Professor
Department of General and GI Surgery
Kathmandu Medical College and Teaching Hospital
Sinamangal, Kathmandu, Nepal

Foreword
Samiran Nundy

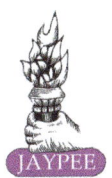

JAYPEE BROTHERS MEDICAL PUBLISHERS
The Health Sciences Publisher
New Delhi | London

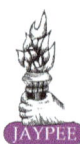

Jaypee Brothers Medical Publishers (P) Ltd

Headquarters

Jaypee Brothers Medical Publishers (P) Ltd
EMCA House, 23/23-B
Ansari Road, Daryaganj
New Delhi 110 002, India
Landline: +91-11-23272143, +91-11-23272703
+91-11-23282021, +91-11-23245672
Email: jaypee@jaypeebrothers.com

Corporate Office

Jaypee Brothers Medical Publishers (P) Ltd
4838/24, Ansari Road, Daryaganj
New Delhi 110 002, India
Phone: +91-11-43574357
Fax: +91-11-43574314
Email: jaypee@jaypeebrothers.com

Overseas Office

JP Medical Ltd
83 Victoria Street, London
SW1H 0HW (UK)
Phone: +44 20 3170 8910
Fax: +44 (0)20 3008 6180
Email: info@jpmedpub.com

Website: www.jaypeebrothers.com
Website: www.jaypeedigital.com

© 2022, Jaypee Brothers Medical Publishers

The views and opinions expressed in this book are solely those of the original contributor(s)/author(s) and do not necessarily represent those of editor(s) of the book.

All rights reserved. No part of this publication may be reproduced, stored or transmitted in any form or by any means, electronic, mechanical, photocopying, recording or otherwise, without the prior permission in writing of the publishers.

All brand names and product names used in this book are trade names, service marks, trademarks or registered trademarks of their respective owners. The publisher is not associated with any product or vendor mentioned in this book.

Medical knowledge and practice change constantly. This book is designed to provide accurate, authoritative information about the subject matter in question. However, readers are advised to check the most current information available on procedures included and check information from the manufacturer of each product to be administered, to verify the recommended dose, formula, method and duration of administration, adverse effects and contraindications. It is the responsibility of the practitioner to take all appropriate safety precautions. Neither the publisher nor the author(s)/editor(s) assume any liability for any injury and/or damage to persons or property arising from or related to use of material in this book.

This book is sold on the understanding that the publisher is not engaged in providing professional medical services. If such advice or services are required, the services of a competent medical professional should be sought.

Every effort has been made where necessary to contact holders of copyright to obtain permission to reproduce copyright material. If any have been inadvertently overlooked, the publisher will be pleased to make the necessary arrangements at the first opportunity. The **CD/DVD-ROM** (if any) provided in the sealed envelope with this book is complimentary and free of cost. **Not meant for sale.**

Inquiries for bulk sales may be solicited at: jaypee@jaypeebrothers.com

Gastrointestinal Surgery Series: Minimal Invasive Hepatobiliary and Pancreas Surgery

First Edition: **2022**

ISBN: 978-93-5465-589-0

Dedicated to

All pioneers in minimal invasive hepato-pancreato-biliary (HPB) surgeons who have pushed their boundaries.

Editorial Board Members

Adarsh Chaudhary MS FRCS
Chairman
Division of GI Surgery, GI Oncology
and Bariatric Surgery
Medanta—The Medicity
Gurugram, Haryana, India

AK Khanna MS MNAMS DSc MBA FACS
FICS FAIS FRSTMH FUWAI FUICC FFIM
Professor
Department of General Surgery
Institute of Medical Sciences
Banaras Hindu University
Varanasi, Uttar Pradesh, India

Arvinder Singh Soin MS FRCS (Edin)
FRCS (Glasgow) FRCS (Transplant Surgery)
Chairman
Medanta Institute of Liver
Transplantation and Regenerative
Medicine, Medanta—The Medicity
Gurugram, Haryana, India

GV Rao MS MAMS FRCS
Director and Chief of Surgical
Gastroenterology and Minimally
Invasive Surgery
Asian Institute of Gastroenterology
Hyderabad, Telangana, India

Ian P Bissett MBChB MD FRACS
Professor, Department of Surgery
School of Medicine
Faculty of Medical and Health Sciences
University of Auckland
Auckland, New Zealand

Manohar Lal Shrestha
MS (Cal) FRCSEd FICS FCPS (Pak) FAIS (Ind)
Professor
(Surgical Gastroenterology and
Colorectal Surgeon)
Department of Surgery
Nepal Medical College and
Teaching Hospital
Attarkhel, Kathmandu, Nepal

Peush Sahni MS PhD
Professor
Department of Gastrointestinal Surgery
and Liver Transplantation
All India Institute of Medical Sciences
New Delhi, India

Piet Pattyn MD PhD
Professor
Department of General and
Digestive Surgery
Ghent University Hospital
Ghent, Belgium

Rahul Khanna
MBBS MS DNB MNAMS FAIS PhD
Professor
Department of General Surgery
Institute of Medical Sciences
Banaras Hindu University
Varanasi, Uttar Pradesh, India

Rajesh Bhojwani MS MCh FCLS
Professor
Department of GI Surgery
Santokba Institute of Digestive Surgical
Sciences (SIDSS)
Jaipur, Rajasthan, India

Roberto Troisi MSc MD PhD FEBS
Full Professor of Surgery
Director HPB, Minimally Invasive
and Robotic Surgery Center
Federico II University, Naples, Italy

Samiran Nundy MCh MA FRCP FRCS
Chairperson of Surgical
Gastroenterology and Liver
Transplantation
Sir Ganga Ram Hospital
New Delhi, India

Sushil Bahadur Rawal MBBS MS
Consultant GI Surgeon
Medicity Hospital
Kathmandu, Nepal

Editorial Board Members

Shailesh V Shrikhande MS MD
Professor
Department of Gastrointestinal and
Hepato-Biliary-Pancreatic Surgery
Tata Memorial Hospital
Mumbai, Maharashtra, India

Vinay Kumaran MS MCh
Professor, Surgical Director, Living Donor
Liver Transplantation
Department of Surgery
Division of Transplant Surgery
West Hospital, Richmond, Virginia, USA

Vijay Kumar Shukla MS MCh FAMS
Professor, Department of General Surgery
Banaras Hindu University
Varanasi, Uttar Pradesh, India

Wim P Ceelen MD PhD FACS
Professor
Department of General
and Digestive Surgery
Ghent University Hospital
Ghent, Belgium

Yves Van Nieuwenhove MD PhD
Professor
Department of General
and Digestive Surgery
Ghent University Hospital
Ghent, Belgium

Contributors

Ammiel Arra
DM (General Surgery) Fellow
Gastrointestinal and HPB Surgical
Oncology, Department of Surgical
Oncology, Tata Memorial Centre
Mumbai, Maharashtra, India

Babu Raja Shrestha MBBS MD
Professor
Department of Anesthesiology
Kathmandu Medical College and
Teaching Hospital
Sinamangal, Kathmandu, Nepal

Brice Gayet MD PhD
Department of Digestive Oncologic
and Metabolic Surgery
Institut Mutualiste Montsouris
Université Paris Descartes
Paris, France

Catherine SC Teh MD FPCS FRCS (Ed)
Chief
Department of Hepatobiliary Pancreatic
Surgery
Makati Medical Centre
St Luke's Medical Centre and National
Kidney and Transplant Institute
Quezon City, Metro Manila, Philippines

Christoph Berchtold MD
Department of General
Visceral and Transplantation
Surgery
University Hospital Heidelberg
Heidelberg, Germany

David Fuks MD PhD
Department of Digestive Oncologic
and Metabolic Surgery
Institut Mutualiste Montsouris,
Université Paris Descartes
Paris, France

Fumiaki Tokito MD
Department of Surgery
Institute of Gastroenterology
Tokyo Women's Medical University
Tokyo, Japan

Giovanni M Garbarino MD
Department of Medical Surgical
Science and Translational Medicine
Sapienza University of Rome
Rome, Italy

Giammauro Berardi MD PhD
Medical Doctor, Department of Surgery
San Camillo Forlanini Hospital of Rome
Rome, Italy

Goro Honda MD PhD FACS
Professor and Chief
Department of Surgery
Institute of Gastroenterology
Tokyo Women's Medical University
Tokyo, Japan

GV Rao MS MAMS FRCS
Director and Chief
Surgical Gastroenterology and
Minimally Invasive Surgery
Asian Institute of Gastroenterology
Hyderabad, Telangana, India

Ioannis Triantafyllidis MD
Department of Digestive, Oncologic and
Metabolic Surgery, Institut Mutualiste
Montsouris, Université Paris Descartes
Paris, France

Katherine M Panganiban
MD FPSGS FPCS
Division of Minimal Invasive and
Robotic Surgery, Institute of Surgery
St Luke's Medical Centre
Quezon City, Metro Manila, Philippines

Contributors

Manish S Bhandare
MS MCh PDF GI and HPB Surgical Oncology
Associate Professor
Department of Gastric
and HPB surgery
Tata Memorial Centre
Mumbai, Maharashtra, India

Marc Beaussier MD PhD
Department of Digestive
Oncologic and Metabolic Surgery
Institut Mutualiste Montsouris
Université Paris Descartes
Paris, France

Masakazu Yamamoto MD PhD
Director
Department of Surgery
Institute of Gastroenterology
Tokyo Women's Medical University
Tokyo, Japan

Maud Neuberg MD
Department of Digestive
Oncologic and Metabolic Surgery
Institut Mutualiste Montsouris
Université Paris Descartes
Paris, France

Naoto Senmaru MD
Department of Gastroenterological
Surgery
Hokkaido University
Graduate School of Medicine
Sapporo, Japan

Rajesh Bhojwani MS MCh FCLS
Professor
Department of GI Surgery
Santokba Institute of Digestive
Surgical Sciences (SIDSS)
Santokba Durlabhji Memorial
Hospital (SDMH)
Jaipur, Rajasthan, India

Roshan Ghimire MBBS MS
Fellowship in HPB and Liver Transplantation
Associate Professor
Department of General and GI Surgery
Kathmandu Medical College and
Teaching Hospital
Sinamangal, Kathmandu, Nepal

Ruchit H Kansaria
MS (General Surgery) MCh
(Surgical Oncology) Fellow
Gastrointestinal and HPB
Surgical Oncology
Tata Memorial Centre
Mumbai, Maharashtra, India

Saseem Poudel MD
Department of Gastroenterological
Surgery
Hokkaido University
Graduate School of Medicine
Sapporo, Japan

Satoshi Hirano MD PhD
Professor
Department of Gastroenterological
Surgery, Hokkaido University
Graduate School of Medicine
Sapporo, Japan

Savio George Barreto MBBS MS PhD
Senior Lecturer in Medicine
Division of Surgery and
Perioperative Medicine
College of Medicine and Public Health
Flinders University, Australia

Shailesh V Shrikhande
MBBS MS MD FRCS (HON)
Deputy Director
Tata Memorial Hospital
Professor of Surgical Oncology
Chief, Hepato-Pancreato-Biliary
Surgical Oncology, Tata Memorial
Centre, Mumbai, Maharashtra, India

Shreeyash Modak MS
Consultant and Surgical Gastroenterologist
Department of Surgical Gastroenterology and Minimally Invasive Surgery
Asian Institute of Gastroenterology
Hyderabad, Telangana, India

Siddhartha Mishra MBBS MS
Clinical Associate
Santokba Institute of Digestive Surgical Sciences (SIDSS)
Santokba Durlabhji Memorial Hospital (SDMH)
Jaipur, Rajasthan, India

Sujan Regmee MBBS MS
Lecturer
Department of General and GI Surgery
Kathmandu Medical College and Teaching Hospital
Sinamangal, Kathmandu, Nepal

Sushila Lama Moktan MBBS MD
Assistant Professor
Department of Anesthesiology
Kathmandu Medical College and Teaching Hospital
Sinamangal, Kathmandu, Nepal

Thilo Hackert MD
Professor
Department of General, Visceral and Transplantation Surgery
University Hospital Heidelberg
Heidelberg, Germany

Vikram Chaudhari DNB (General Surgery)
DNB (Surgical Gastroenterology)
PDF (GI and HPB Surgical Oncology)
Associate Professor
Department of Surgical Oncology
Tata Memorial Centre
Mumbai, Maharashtra, India

Yoshikuni Kawaguchi MD PhD
Department of Digestive Oncologic and Metabolic Surgery
Institute Mutualiste Montsouris
Université Paris Descartes
Paris, France

Yugal Limbu MBBS MS
Lecturer, Department of General and GI Surgery, Kathmandu Medical College and Teaching Hospital
Sinamangal, Kathmandu, Nepal

Yusuke Ome MD PhD FACS
Department of Surgery
Institute of Gastroenterology
Tokyo Women's Medical University
Tokyo, Japan

Foreword

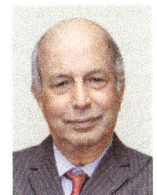

Who would have thought that such a book discussing the different aspects of such complex, innovative and the most contemporary surgical procedures would come out of a small country like Nepal. It is indeed a remarkable achievement, and I am proud to have been asked to write the foreword.

Drs Dhiresh Kumar Maharjan and Prabin Bikram Thapa have gathered 34 surgeons from eight countries (Australia, France, Germany, Japan, India, Italy and the Philippines as well as their own colleagues in Nepal) to describe not only how to perform major procedures on the gallbladder, liver, bile ducts and pancreas but also place them in our present context. Thus, not only, for instance, are the techniques for robotic pancreaticoduodenectomy discussed, but also there are chapters on anesthesia, how to control intraoperative bleeding, the use of indocyanine green and starting laparoscopic hepatectomy in a low volume center. The well-known advantages of minimally invasive procedures are their cosmetic result, the lower blood loss and shorter hospital stay, and faster recovery compared to open operations. There is also evidence that during operations for carcinoma the outcomes are similar to the open technique regarding margins and lymph node retrieval.

However, I, who only performs open operations, must add a word of caution here. Lord Cohen of Birkenhead, the distinguished British physician once said that the 'Feasibility of an operation is not an indication for it'. Any new procedure should be carefully evaluated regarding whether it is safe, effective, and affordable and the decision to perform it should be based on hard evidence. In fact, there are very few prospective randomized studies comparing minimally invasive and open surgery (there have been some American and Dutch trials which were terminated because of the higher mortality of these procedures) and apart from cholecystectomy and distal pancreatectomy I cannot think of any other operation which has become firmly established. The results of any surgical operation not only depend on surgical expertise but also on patient selection. Thus, publications on minimally invasive surgery are usually authored by those very experienced in the field who have generally performed procedures on thin patients with early disease. There is also a publication bias because even these surgeons will tell the world about their results if they are good. Those who have had major morbidity and mortality are hardly likely to write or speak about them.

Thus, although I think that minimally invasive surgery is the future before it is more widely adopted, especially in developing countries, it should be carefully evaluated on whether it is safe (probably not), effective (yes in experienced hands) and affordable (no). We must remember that these complex procedures all have a very steep learning curve, and some have suggested that before embarking on them at least 30-50 procedures should have been performed under supervision. This is a rather tall order and not feasible for most surgeons in our countries.

Nevertheless, the Editors have done us a great service in producing a book which tells us what is possible using these techniques and should be congratulated for their efforts. Everyone interested in the future of hepatobiliary and pancreatic surgery should read this book.

Samiran Nundy MCH MA FRCP FRCS
Chairperson of Surgical Gastroenterology
and Liver Transplantation
Sir Ganga Ram Hospital
New Delhi, India

Preface

Means of acquisition of knowledge never fades, but changes with time, so do our perseverance for academic excellence. Since the conception of the handbook entitled "Gastrointestinal Surgery Series," "Pancreas and Hepatobiliary Surgery" in 2018, we were lagging in widely accepted minimal invasive hepato-pancreato-biliary (HPB) surgery as there had been rapidly evolving surgical techniques.

This book provides recent advances in the minimal invasive surgery from laparoscopic to the robotic approach of liver resection and approaches of minimal invasive Whipple operation, both laparoscopic and robotic.

This book would be an armamentarium mainly for surgical residents and young laparoscopic surgeon trying to set up laparoscopic HPB surgery and troubleshooting problems tips while performing it.

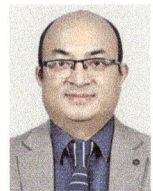 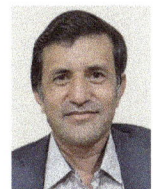

Dhiresh Kumar Maharjan   **Prabin Bikram Thapa**

Acknowledgments

We would like to acknowledge Prof Suman Kumar Shrestha, Dr Roshan Ghimire, Dr Anuj Parajuli, Dr Uttam Laudari, Dr Santosh Shrestha, Dr Yugal Limbu, Dr Sujan Regmi, and our junior faculties. We would like to thank Mr Drishant Maharjan for his assistance in illustration.

Contents

1. **Anesthetic Viewpoints in Laparoscopic Liver Resection** 1
   Babu Raja Shrestha, Sushila Lama Moktan

2. **Intraoperative Bleeding Control during Laparoscopic Liver Resections** 6
   Ioannis Triantafyllidis, Maud Neuberg, Yoshikuni Kawaguchi, Marc Beaussier, Brice Gayet, David Fuks

3. **Initiating Laparoscopic Hepatectomy in Low-volume Center** 14
   Saseem Poudel, Naoto Senmaru, Satoshi Hirano

4. **Role of Indocyanine Green in Laparoscopic Liver Surgery** 20
   Katherine M Panganiban, Catherine SC Teh

5. **Laparoscopic Right Hepatectomy** 32
   Fumiaki Tokito, Yusuke Ome, Goro Honda, Masakazu Yamamoto

6. **Minimal Invasive Treatment for Colorectal Liver Metastases** 37
   Giovanni M Garbarino, Giammauro Berardi

7. **Minimally Invasive Surgery in Gallbladder Carcinoma** 50
   Yugal Limbu, Sujan Regmee, Roshan Ghimire

8. **Changing Trends in Minimal Invasive Pancreatic Surgery** 57
   Savio George Barreto

9. **Laparoscopic Pancreaticoduodenectomy** 65
   Siddhartha Mishra, Rajesh Bhojwani

10. **Initiating Robotic Pancreaticoduodenectomy** 78
    Ruchit H Kansaria, Manish S Bhandare, Vikram Chaudhari, Ammiel Arra, Shailesh V Shrikhande

11. **Minimally Invasive Distal Pancreatectomy** 105
    Christoph Berchtold, Thilo Hackert

12. **Minimally Invasive Approach to Chronic Pancreatitis** 115
    Shreeyash Modak, GV Rao

    Index 123

CHAPTER 1

Anesthetic Viewpoints in Laparoscopic Liver Resection

Babu Raja Shrestha, Sushila Lama Moktan

INTRODUCTION

Major abdominal surgery leads to major physiological deviations. Every anesthetic endeavor should be directed to preserve the physiological balance during and after the surgical interventions associated with inherent risks of bleeding, hemodynamic fluctuations, fluid shifts, coagulopathy, and pulmonary and renal impairments including postoperative hepatic failure.

Era of laparoscopic liver resection demands meticulous anesthetic patient care perioperatively. Laparoscopic liver resection unless fine-tuned with anesthetic manipulation, the untoward effects are accentuated and even inevitable. The advent of this minimal invasive hepatic resection technique mandates anesthetic counterparts to stay in close touch with the changing physiological parameters during surgery. Growing surgical expertise and anesthetic experiences have allowed several limitations to overcome since the first laparoscopic liver resection in 1991.[1]

Preoperative evaluation and assessment should be tailored according to the existing liver function status and comorbidities. Detailed laboratory investigations and risk stratifications warrant preoperative optimization and perioperative planning. Liver function reserve is evaluated, and the candidate is categorized as per Child–Pugh classification. This aids to determine extent, possibility, and prognostication of liver resection.

CHOICE OF ANESTHESIA

Liver-friendly general anesthesia with endotracheal intubation under controlled ventilation is key in laparoscopic liver resection.

For best perioperative analgesia, thoracic epidural catheter placement is widely employed and maximum care is exercised during, and at the time of epidural catheter removal. Epidural analgesics has been claimed to be immune-protective.[2] Moreover, other benefits such as reduced thromboembolism, preservation of respiratory function, and early return of gastrointestinal mobility are in favor of thoracic epidural placement.[3] Postresection international normalized ratio (INR) should be <1.3 prior to epidural catheter removal. Unless the INR is normalized, fresh-frozen plasma transfusion, injection vitamin K is indicated before catheter removal.[4]

An important issue with regards to thoracic epidural in laparoscopic liver resection is fear of acute kidney injury (AKI) on the background of sympathetic truncation, peripheral vasodilatation, compromised central venous pressure (CVP) during liver resection, miser crystalloid infusion at times during parenchymal resection, and compromised hemodynamics in condition of probable torrential intraoperative bleeding.

Another effective alternative for analgesia is single shot intrathecal morphine (200-300 μg) with bupivacaine along with premedication of gabapentin. The extent of analgesia provided by this mode is comparable to epidural analgesia for early postoperative period of 48 hours.[5]

Point to Note

Perioperative opioid use might retard gastrointestinal function as liver resection might increase bioavailability of opioids due to reduced drug metabolism and subsequent accumulation. This demands vigilant postoperative respiratory monitoring to protect the patients from possible respiratory depression.

SOME ISSUES ON COAGULATION

Postoperative coagulopathy after laparoscopic liver resection is dependent on various factors such as previous hepatic liver dysfunction, prothrombin time (PT), INR, platelet function, extent of liver resection and remnant functional hepatic volume, duration of surgery, volume of blood transfusion, and extent of ischemia reperfusion injury.

Foundation resource management for laparoscopic liver resection enthusiasts in countries such as Nepal is arrangement of viscoelastic coagulation testing arrangement. This facility offers evaluation of both procoagulant activity and endogenous anticoagulation. Viscoelastic coagulation study demonstrates normal, hypercoagulable, and clot strength following laparoscopic liver resection enabling appropriate measures accordingly. Factors such as acidosis, hypocalcemia, and hypothermia must be regularly monitored in order not to amplify coagulation disorders.[6]

WHAT ANESTHESIOLOGISTS NEED TO DO TO MINIMIZE INTRAOPERATIVE BLEEDING DURING LAPAROSCOPIC LIVER RESECTION?

- Keep the patient in head-up, reverse Trendelenburg position to unload the vascular beds during bleeding.
- Increase carbon dioxide pneumoperitoneum pressure from 12 to 15-16 mm Hg. This helps compress vascular weeping from vessels other than inferior vena cava.
- Restrict intravenous crystalloid infusion down to 1 mL/kg/h during liver parenchymal resection period.
- Maintain CVP <5 mm Hg **(Fig. 1)**.[7]

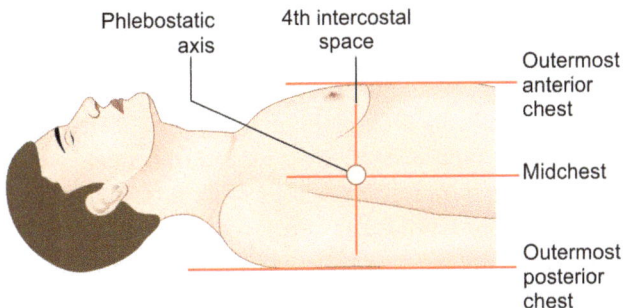

Fig. 1: Central venous pressure (CVP) monitoring keeping at phlebostatic axis.

Hepatic valve-less veins might allow backflow of blood during hepatic inflow occlusion, thus lowering CVP significantly decreases bleeding. In order not to increase effects of bleeding, anesthesiologists may consider preoperative therapy of erythropoietin and intraoperative use of warming blankets and warm fluids to check hypothermia.

PITFALLS AND CHALLENGES OF LOW CENTRAL VENOUS PRESSURE IN LAPAROSCOPIC LIVER RESECTION

The first basic need is to note down the individual CVP in the beginning of the surgery. This allows us to consider the factors that might elevate or lower CVP. Risks of lowering CVP predispose patient to hemodynamic instability—decrease cardiac output, decrease mean arterial pressure, and decrease perfusion pressure to the vital organs.

These after-effects of minimized CVP are further accentuated due to the carbon dioxide pneumoperitoneum compressing the major intra-abdominal vasculatures. However, these conditions reduce the distension of the central veins aiding hepatic dissection.

All the maneuvers employed during bleeding are not in favor of maintaining hemodynamics and add on further challenges to anesthesiologists. This demands expertise, skill, and vigilance from anesthetic counterpart. Fluid restriction head-up position, epidural, nitroglycerin, and diuretics might help reduce CVP. Besides, positioning patient in left lateral tilt keeps hepatic veins superior to the inferior vena cava and venous bleeding is decreased during parenchymal dissection.

Preexisting conditions such as right ventricular pressure overload due to pulmonary artery hypertension (PAH), tricuspid valve pathology, auto-positive end-expiratory pressure (PEEP) from pulmonary pathology might change the actual CVP readings. CVP recording at mid-axillary point should also be well fixed for continuous CVP tracing. Stroke volume variation (SVV) monitoring is another monitoring technique where CVP measure loses its validity.[8] Compression on liver and diaphragm by multiple surgical pads may be another point to note if CVP is persistently high despite all above-mentioned techniques. Intermittent total hepatic inflow clamping is another widely adopted technique for this purpose to control bleeding (Pringle technique).[9]

Laparoscopic liver resection poses another serious condition such as probability of gas embolism (incidence 0.2–1.5%).[10] The risk of venous gas embolism during laparoscopic liver resection is likely when favorable condition of gas entrainment into venous system is created by increasing CO_2 pneumoperitoneum in the background of lowered down CVP with no intention of minimizing bleeding during liver resection. However, despite positive pressure gradient between CVP and intra-abdominal pressure (IAP) (CVP > IAP), gas embolism can still occur due to volume and rate of CO_2 insufflation.[11,12]

This raises a question that laparoscopic liver resection might have different CVP target than in open liver resection as low CVP demanded by operating surgeon might increasingly predispose CO_2 gas embolism when IAP-CVP gradient is continuously positive, with negative suctioning effect transferred from the thoracic cavity. The practical solution to this issue is prevention and earlier recognition of gas embolism by comprehensive monitoring system such as transesophageal echocardiography (TEE), precordial Doppler, and capnography.

INTRAVENOUS FLUID

It is strongly recommended to use balanced crystalloid (Plasma-Lyte) and avoid 0.9% normal saline to avoid postoperative hyperchloremia and renal dysfunction.[13]

POSTOPERATIVE ISSUES

Closer monitoring of liver enzymes, coagulogram, and renal function is the key to early recognition and treatment. Early enteral nutrition, electrolyte correction, and avoidance of hepatotoxic agents expedites restoration of liver functionality.

CONCLUSION

Laparoscopic liver resection demands meticulous understanding of ongoing physiology. This allows anesthetic modification and techniques which create favorable surgical field and helps overcome untoward effects with vigilance, communication in the team for better operative outcomes, and subsequent patient recovery.

REFERENCES

1. Guro H, Cho JY, Han HS, Yoon YS, Choi YR, Periyasami M. Current status of laparoscopic liver resection for hepatocellular carcinoma. Clin Mol Hepatol. 2016;22(2):212-8.

2. Clavien PA, Petrowsky H, DeOliveria ML, Graf R. strategies for safer liver surgery and partial liver transplantation. N Engl J Med. 2007;356(15):1545-59.
3. Siniscalchi A, Gamberini L, Bardi T, Laici C, Gamberini E, Francirsi L, et al. Role of epidural anesthesia in fast track liver resection protocol for cirrhotic patients- results after three years of practice. World J Hepatol. 2016;8(26):1097-104.
4. Elterman KG, Xiong Z. Coagulation profile changes and safety of epidural analgesia after hepatectomy: a retrospective study. J Anesth. 2015;29(3):367-72.
5. De Pietri L, Siniscalchi A, Reggiani A, Masetti M, Begliomini B, Gazzi M, et al. The use of intrathecal morphine morphine for postoperative pain relief after liver resection: a comparison with epidural analgesia. Anesth Analg 2006;102(4):1157-63.
6. Mallet SV, Sugavanam A, Krzanicki DA, Patel S, Broomhead RH, Davidson BR, et.al. Alterations in coagulation following major liver resection. Anesthesia. 2016;71(6):657-68.
7. Zhu P, Lau WY, Chen YF, Zyang BX, Huang ZY, Zyang ZW, et al. Randomized clinical trial comparing infrahepatic inferior vena cava clamping with low central venous pressure in complex liver resections involving the Pringle manoeuvre. Br J Surg. 2012;99(6):781-8.
8. Katiguchi K, Gotohda N, Yamamoto H, Takahashi S, Konishi M, Hayashi R. A comparative study of intraoperative fluid management using stroke volume variation in liver resection. Int Surg. 2018;103(3-4):199-206.
9. Selzer N, Rudiger H, Graf R, Clavien PA. Protective strategies against ischemic injury of the liver. Gastroenterology. 2003;125(3):917-36.
10. Schmandra TC, Mierdl S, Bauer H, Gutt C, Hanisch E. Transesophageal echocardiography shows high risk of gas embolism during laparoscopic hepatic resection under carbon dioxide pneumoperitoneum. Br J Surg. 2002;89(7):870-6.
11. Jones RM, Moulton CE, Hardy KJ. Central venous pressure and its effect on blood loss during liver resection. Br J Surg. 1998;85(8):1058-60.
12. Giordano C, Gravenstein N, Rice M. What is the optimal CVP to minimize risk in patients undergoing laparoscopic hepatectomy? Circulation. 2013;28(1):8.
13. Shin WJ, Kim YK, Bang JY, Cho SK, Han SM, Hwang GS. Lactate and liver function tests after living donor right hepatectomy: a comparison of solutions with and without lactate. Acta Anesthesiol Scand. 2011;55(5):558-64.

CHAPTER

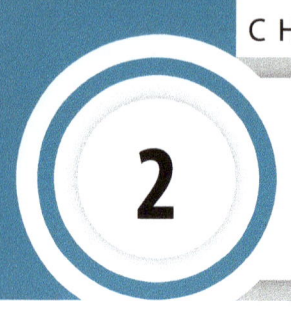

Intraoperative Bleeding Control during Laparoscopic Liver Resections

*Ioannis Triantafyllidis, Maud Neuberg, Yoshikuni Kawaguchi,
Marc Beaussier, Brice Gayet, David Fuks*

■ INTRODUCTION

Laparoscopic hepatectomy gained increased popularity during the last decades due to the technical refinements and accumulation of experience and expertise. Recent series of major liver resections demonstrate postoperative mortality rates of 0.7–2.6%,[1,2] while morbidity ranges from 1 to 56.4%.[1,3] Although, blood loss accompanied by increased blood transfusions remains the Achilles' heel of laparoscopic liver surgery resulting in a higher rate of recurrence and lower survival after resection of colorectal liver metastases and hepatocellular carcinoma.[4,5] It is well documented that there is less intraoperative blood loss in laparoscopic approach when compared to open hepatectomy. It is more likely that the main reasons for reduced blood loss during laparoscopic liver resections are the increased intra-abdominal pressure due to the pneumoperitoneum, the precision afforded by the magnified view that allows surgeons to undertake precise manipulations, the development of new transection devices, the maintenance of low central venous pressure during transection, and the facilitation of inflow and outflow control.[6-9] However, bleeding control during laparoscopic hepatectomy is more technically demanding than during open hepatectomy, but still remains the cornerstone of a successful operation.[10]

■ BASIC SURGICAL TECHNIQUES

The basic surgical techniques that we use for luteinizing hormone (LH) are described elsewhere.[11-13] Briefly, anesthetized patients are positioned in low lithotomy, with the hips abducted and knees flexed (French position). A 12-mm trocar is introduced through the anterior abdominal wall near the umbilicus to accommodate the camera. Another 12-mm trocar is placed high in the right hypochondrium for intraoperative ultrasonography and vascular stapling. Three or four additional 5-mm operative ports are also placed. A tape is placed around the hepatoduodenal ligament to allow inflow to be occluded, but intermittent inflow occlusion (Pringle maneuver) is used only in case of massive and/or persistent bleeding.[10,11] Parenchymal transection is performed with bipolar forceps (Micro France CEVBG134; Medtronic, Minneapolis, MN, USA) and an ultrasonic cutting and coagulating device (Thunderbeat; Olympus). After parenchymal transection, the resected specimen is placed in a plastic bag and retrieved whole through a small incision which was normally made in the lower abdomen. Fibrin glue or a carrier-bound fibrin sealant can be placed on the raw surface. Drains are placed only if there is concern about increased risk of postoperative bleeding or bile leak.[10-14]

NONOPERATIVE METHODS OF MINIMIZING BLOOD LOSS

Intra-abdominal pressure is maintained between 10 and 12 mm Hg and raised to 15–16 mm Hg if there is massive bleeding not arising from the inferior vena cava. During parenchymal transection, the rate of intravenous fluid administration is decreased and maintained as low as 1 mL/kg/h, and the central venous pressure is maintained ≤5 cmH$_2$O to facilitate the hemostatic effect of the pneumoperitoneum on the transection surface.[10]

Apart from pneumoperitoneum which is likely to reduce bleeding from the hepatic veins, placement of the patient in the reverse Trendelenburg position should help decrease the venous pressure and improve exposure by gravitationally shifting visceral structures away from the liver hilum, in cases deemed to be difficult at the preoperative assessment. Other conceptual changes include the superior and lateral approaches with or without the use of intercostal or transthoracic trocars. For these approaches, the patient is placed in the left lateral decubitus position. The left lateral decubitus position or even the prone position offers better exposure of the right posterior segments and lifts the right hepatic vein higher than the vena cava to reduce hepatic venous bleeding.[10,15]

TECHNIQUES FOR BLEEDING CONTROL

General Considerations

The superficial 2 cm of the liver parenchyma contains small vessels that can easily be secured. Larger vessels, such as hepatic or portal veins, are located deeper, while inflow pedicles are more solid and surrounded by a Glisson sheath. As a result, dealing with deeper transection necessitates identification of the vessels and selective ligation. In general, vessels with diameter <5 mm are coagulated and transected using an energy device or bipolar diathermy or closed by clips. Vessels with diameter 5–10 mm are ligated with plastic locking clips (Hem-o-lok, Teleflex Medical) and then divided, especially in cases of patients with extensive arteriosclerosis. Laparoscopic linear staplers (Endo GIA, Covidien; Echelon Endopath, Ethicon Endo-Surgery) are used for larger vessels. The stapler can be applied to segmental portal pedicles or to isolated large portal or hepatic veins.

Effective transection of the liver parenchyma with minimal blood loss is of paramount importance for a safe laparoscopic hepatectomy. However, continuous suction interferes with pneumoperitoneum pressure, and bleeding control is more technically demanding in comparison with open hepatectomy.

When operating laparoscopically, it is not possible to compress the whole liver, to lift the liver to reduce venous pressure, or achieve a full range of movement of the forceps. Furthermore, hypertension, neoadjuvant chemotherapy, major hepatectomy, and resection of posterosuperior segments are associated with increased blood loss.[10] After all, intraoperative bleeding control is key to successful liver surgery. To achieve this goal, the hepatopancreatobiliary (HPB) laparoscopic surgeon has various options in his armamentarium.

Inflow Occlusion Technique

The Pringle inflow occlusion technique is performed whenever necessary for the control of torrential and/or persistent bleeding. We apply it intermittently, with 15–20 minutes of occlusion alternating with 5 minutes of reperfusion. For patients without liver cirrhosis, the occlusion time can be extended, if needed. In addition, segmental or subsegmental portal pedicles are dissected and occluded/divided prior to parenchymal transection when the corresponding segment or subsegment is resected.

Removal of Bipolar Forceps while Continuing to Apply Current

In our department (Institut Mutualiste Montsouris, Paris-France), the primary method for hemostasis is the use of bipolar forceps. These should be removed from a point of bleeding with the current still applied. If the application of current ceases before the forceps are withdrawn, the coagulated tissues adherent to the tips are also removed and bleeding is likely to recur.

Replacement of Bipolar Forceps

After bipolar coagulation, burnt tissues adhering to the tips of the bipolar forceps will reduce the efficiency of coagulation **(Figs. 1A and B)**. Bipolar forceps with adherent tissue should be replaced immediately with cleaner ones when necessary. For this purpose, at least two identical pairs of hemostatic instruments should be available during surgery.

Preservation or Increase of Intra-abdominal Pressure

The first step to control bleeding is to apply gentle pressure to the liver surface with the forceps, allowing the point of bleeding to be identified while blood is aspirated by suction. Suction should be applied sparingly to avoid reductions in intra-abdominal pressure. Low intra-abdominal pressure may cause a surge in bleeding, making achieving hemostasis even more challenging. Intra-abdominal pressure may rapidly decline to <5 mm Hg if

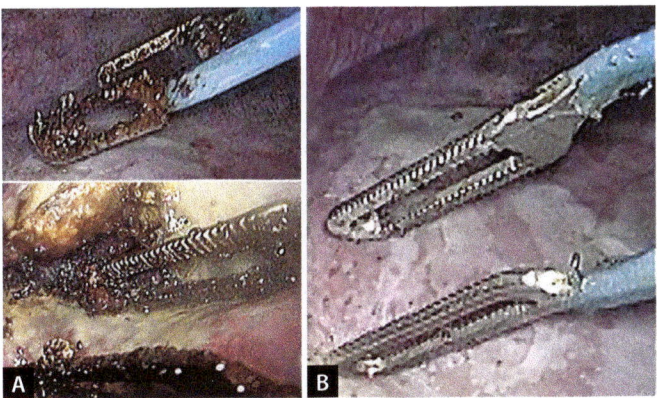

Figs. 1A and B: (A) Tips of the bipolar forceps with adherent coagulated tissue; (B) Tip of the bipolar forceps before performing coagulation.

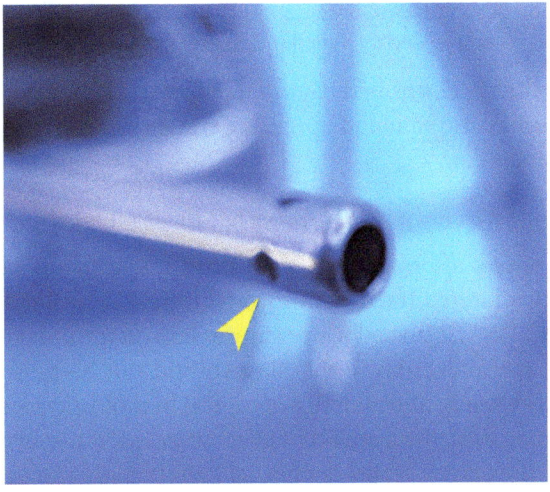

Fig. 2: Suction catheter tip with only one row of holes (arrowhead).

care is not taken when suction is used. We employ a suction catheter with a small number and area of holes at the tip (aspiration-lavage tip; Medtronic) to avoid this potential complication **(Fig. 2)**.

In cases of severe bleeding, increasing the pneumoperitoneum pressure to 16–20 mm Hg and decreasing the airway pressure by a brief pause in the artificial ventilation are maneuvers that can be used to decrease back-bleeding.[15]

Bipolar Coagulation with Simultaneous Compression of the Liver Parenchyma

Undertaking bipolar coagulation while simultaneously compressing the liver parenchyma with forceps or a suction catheter **(Fig. 3)** can be effective when

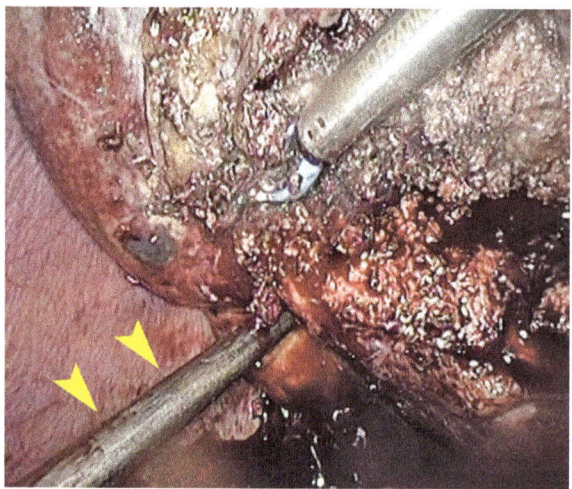

Fig. 3: Bipolar coagulation was performed while the surface of the liver was compressed by a suction catheter (arrowheads).

bleeding is not fully controlled. Gentle compression with forceps reduces pressure in the hepatic vein and optimizes contact between the device's tips and the bleeding point.

Bipolar Coagulation and Placement of Fibrillar Oxidized Cellulose

If bleeding persists after attempts to control it with coagulation, a small amount of fibrillar oxidized cellulose (Surgical Fibrillar; Ethicon Inc, Cincinnati, OH, USA) is placed with compression on the point of subsequent oozing. Further transection of the liver should not be performed unless hemostasis has been confirmed. Use of topical hemostatic agents is sensible in cases of oozing from the transected liver surface. The use of carrier-bound fibrin sealant in various series decreased significantly the time needed to achieve hemostasis, but did not decrease red blood cell transfusions, postoperative collections, and bile leaks.[1]

Bleeding of Peripheral Portal Pedicle

Massive bleeding at the stump of a peripheral portal pedicle, which is accidentally injured before its exposure, can be controlled by a combination of bipolar coagulation with simultaneous compression of the liver parenchyma and preservation of intra-abdominal pressure. In some cases, the Pringle maneuver or clamping of the hepatic artery might also be helpful.

Bleeding Directly from the Hepatic Vein: Instantaneous (Single-shot) Bipolar Coagulation

Instantaneous (single-shot) coagulation with bipolar forceps can be an effective means of addressing bleeding from small holes in the wall of the hepatic vein. Relatively large holes in the hepatic vein may be closed with nonabsorbable suture after compression at the point of bleeding with gauze and/or vascular clamping.

Introduction of a Gauze through a Hand-assisted System at the Beginning of the Procedure

A gauze may be introduced using a hand-assisted system before parenchymal transection in case of anticipation of massive hemorrhage. This system allows surgeons to apply pressure on the point of bleeding with the gauze using his or her hands, providing a rapid and stable means of controlling bleeding.

Conversion to an Open Approach

Conversion to an open approach is required when efforts to control bleeding laparoscopically have failed. Laparotomy decreases the intra-abdominal pressure, so may provoke further massive bleeding and hemodynamic instability. The risk of bleeding during parenchymal transection on the liver surface is considered to be lower than transection deeper within the liver.

Supplementary Technique: Bleeding Control Using a Monopolar Electrode with Saline Irrigation (Not Routinely Used)

Bleeding from the hepatic vein or the cut surface of the liver may be controlled using a monopolar electrode irrigated with saline (IO-Advance electrode®; AMCO Inc, Tokyo, Japan). The presence of saline reduces the current density and avoids carbonization of the tissue and therefore re-bleeding caused by accidental removal of burnt tissue on the coagulated cut surface.

■ CONCLUSION

The crucial technical points of laparoscopic bleeding control are to utilize properly hemostatic devices to undertake meticulously hemostatic procedures by coordinating the use of forceps or a suction catheter with another hand and to use suction sparingly so as not to decrease intra-abdominal pressure. Laparoscopic suturing skills are essential for laparoscopic hepatectomy as the First and Second International Consensus Conference on Laparoscopic Liver Resections recommended,[1,15,16] and staplers are reliable for bleeding control of a broad pedicle of tissue.[17] Bipolar forceps are commonly used for bleeding control at our institution and essentially required for surgical techniques 2, 7, and 8. However, other techniques can be applied with different hemostatic devices. Namely, inflow occlusion (surgical technique 1), preparation of two identical pairs of hemostatic instruments (surgical technique 3), preservation of intra-abdominal pressure during aspiration of blood (surgical technique 4), compression of the liver parenchyma (surgical technique 5), placement of fibrillar oxidized cellulose (surgical technique 6), a gauze introduction through a hand-assisted system (surgical technique 9), and decision to conversion (surgical technique 10) are expected to be useful when using other hemostatic devices.

REFERENCES

1. Brustia R, Granger B, Scatton O. An update on topical haemostatic agents in liver surgery: systematic review and meta analysis. Hepatobiliary Pancreat Sci. 2016;23(10):609-21.
2. Dokmak S, Ftériche FS, Borscheid R, Cauchy F, Farges O, Belghiti J. 2012 Liver resections in the 21st century: we are far from zero mortality. HPB (Oxford). 2013;15(11):908-15.
3. Page AJ, Gani F, Crowley KT, Lee KH, Grant MC, Zavadsky TL, et al. Patient outcomes and provider perceptions following implementation of a standardized perioperative care pathway for open liver resection. Br J Surg. 2016;103(5):564-71.
4. Stephenson KR, Steinberg SM, Hughes KS, Vetto JT, Sugarbaker PH, Chang AE. Perioperative blood transfusions are associated with decreased time to recurrence and decreased survival after resection of colorectal liver metastases. Ann Surg. 1988;208(6):679-87.
5. Katz SC, Shia J, Liau KH, Gonen M, Ruo L, Jarnagin WR, et al. Operative blood loss independently predicts recurrence and survival after resection of hepatocellular carcinoma. Ann Surg. 2009;249(4):617-23.
6. Tranchart H, O'Rourke N, Van Dam R, Gaillard M, Lainas P, Sugioka A, et al. Bleeding control during laparoscopic liver resection: a review of literature. J Hepatobiliary Pancreat Sci. 2015;22(5):371-8.
7. Tympa A, Theodoraki K, Tsaroucha A, Arkadopoulos N, Vassiliou I, Smyrniotis V. Anesthetic considerations in hepatectomies under hepatic vascular control. HPB Surg. 2012;2012:720754.
8. Nguyen KT, Gamblin TC, Geller DA. World review of laparoscopic liver resection-2,804 patients. Ann Surg. 2009;250:831-41.
9. Soubrane O, Schwarz L, Cauchy F, Perotto LO, Brustia R, Bernard D, et al. A conceptual technique for laparoscopic right hepatectomy based on facts and oncologic principles: the caudal approach. Ann Surg. 2015;261(6):1226-31.
10. Kawaguchi Y, Nomi T, Fuks D, Mal F, Kokudo N, Gayet B. Hemorrhage control for laparoscopic hepatectomy: technical details and predictive factors for intraoperative blood loss. Surg Endosc. 2016;30(6):2543-51.
11. Vibert E, Perniceni T, Levard H, Denet C, Shahri NK, Gayet B. Laparoscopic liver resection. Br J Surg. 2006;93(1):67-72.
12. Gayet B, Cavaliere D, Vibert E, Perniceni T, Levard H, Denet C, et al. Totally laparoscopic right hepatectomy. Am J Surg. 2007;194(5):685-9.
13. Gumbs AA, Gayet B. Adopting Gayet's techniques of totally laparoscopic liver surgery in the United States. Liver Cancer. 2013;2(1):5-15.
14. Ishizawa T, Zuker NB, Conrad C, Lei HJ, Ciacio O, Kokudo N, et al. Using a 'no drain' policy in 342 laparoscopic hepatectomies: which factors predict failure. HPB (Oxford). 2013;16(5):494-9.

15. Wakabayashi G, Cherqui D, Geller DA, Buell JF, Kaneko H, Han HS, et al. Recommendations for laparoscopic liver resection: a report from the second international consensus conference held in Morioka. Ann Surg. 2015;261(4):619-29.
16. Buell JF, Cherqui D, Geller DA, O'Rourke N, Iannitti D, Dagher I, et al. The international position on laparoscopic liver surgery. Ann Surg. 2009; 250(5):825-830.
17. Abu Hilal M, Underwood T, Taylor MG, Hamdan K, Elberm H, Pearce NW. Bleeding and hemostasis in laparoscopic liver surgery. Surg Endosc. 2010; 24(3):572-7.

CHAPTER

Initiating Laparoscopic Hepatectomy in Low-volume Center

3

Saseem Poudel, Naoto Senmaru, Satoshi Hirano

INTRODUCTION

Reich et al.[1] reported the first laparoscopic partial hepatectomy in 1991 and laparoscopic left lateral sectionectomy was reported independently by Azagras et al.[2] and Kaneko et al.[3] in 1996. Since then, laparoscopic hepatectomy has been widely adopted in developed countries especially for partial hepatectomies and left lateral sectionectomy. Meta-analyses have shown laparoscopic hepatectomies to have less blood loss and complications, shorter hospital stay with similar or longer operation time compared to open hepatectomies.[4,5] It allows for magnified view of various anatomy, especially for the liver inside the ribcage. Pneumoperitoneum helps reduce the intraoperative bleeding. However, it should be noted that the studies published are from high-volume centers with expertise in both laparoscopic surgery and hepatobiliary surgery. There are concerns of cost, technical difficulty, and lack of overview that need to be addressed while adopting laparoscopic hepatectomies in low-volume centers, especially in context of developing countries.

COST

Laparoscopic hepatectomy requires many energy devices to maintain hemostasis. It is not unusual for both the surgeon and assistant using as many as three energy devices at the same time. Energy devices commonly used are: Laparoscopic Clarity Ultrasonic Surgical Aspirator System (CUSA®), laparoscopic ultrasonic sears (Harmonic Scarpel®), advanced bipolar vessel sealing device (Ligasure®), and advanced coagulation modes in cautery. All of these have initial setup cost as well as the cost of disposable units used in each operation. Laparoscopic hepatectomy also requires laparoscopic ultrasound device to locate the tumor and vessels as well as staplers to divide major vessels in major hepatectomies.

A study by Cipriani et al.[6] showed that these costs are however offset by shorter hospital stay, lower rate of transfusion, less investigation, and lower severe complications and readmission. However, it should be noted that the study is from western scenario where the cost of hospital stay and instrument differ from the cost in Nepal. Also, the study has reported that the cost becomes higher with conversion cases. So, it is important to first select the cases with a less probability of conversion.

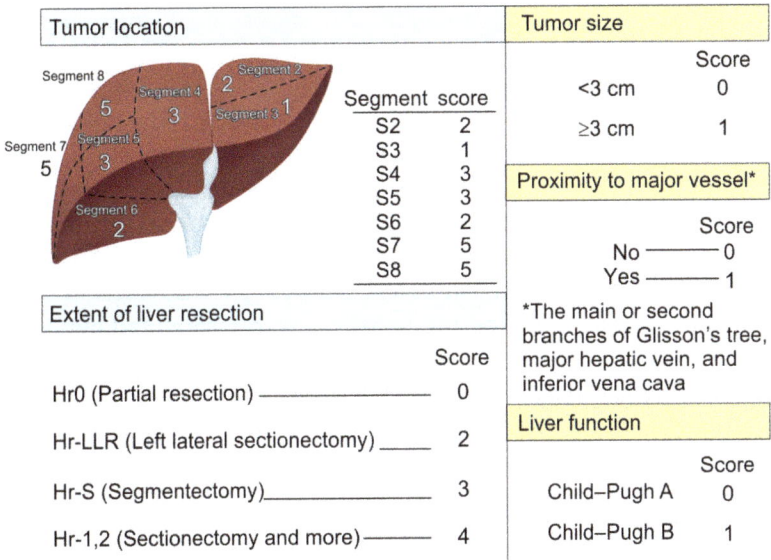

Fig. 1: Technical difficulty scoring system by Ban et al.[7]

TECHNICAL DIFFICULTY

All segments of the liver are not equally accessible and suited for laparoscopic hepatectomy. Ban et al.[7] came up with the technical difficulty scoring system based on the location of the tumor, extent of liver resection, size of the tumor, proximity to major vessels, and liver function **(Fig. 1)**. For the surgeons starting laparoscopic liver resections and with the experience of <10 cases of laparoscopic liver resection, it is recommended to start with liver resection with low difficulty such as simple and small partial hepatectomies in Section 3. Anterior and lateral segments are more accessible laparoscopically than posterior and superior segments. Lesions in these regions can be a good starting point for surgeons starting with laparoscopic hepatectomy.

As the surgeon who can consistently perform "low difficulty" liver resection cases with experience of 10–50 liver resections can move to intermediate difficulty liver resection cases such as left lateral sectionectomy. This has relatively a small transection plane which lies caudal to cranial direction making it easily accessible with traditional laparoscopic port placement. For surgeons who can consistently perform intermediate difficulty level laparoscopic liver resection cases and with the experience of >50 laparoscopic liver resection cases can attempt high difficulty cases such as simple hemihepatectomy. The study also recognizes difficulty score of 10 as the technical limitation of current laparoscopic surgery.

Laparoscopic hepatectomy has a long learning curve of 45–75 cases for major hepatectomy.[8-10] It is recommended to be attempted in high-volume centers with dedicated teams. Even with the dedicated team complications can occur if the technical limitations are not taken into consideration. In one case series in Japan, which has defined the adaptation of laparoscopic liver resection in the country, a team performed 92 cases in three and a half year. However, 58 cases were complex cases and they had eight mortality including four mortality in the first year itself. This led to an external investigation which found that they had not performed adequate preoperative evaluations on liver function. Discussions among the groups were inadequate and external evaluations were also inadequate. The investigation panel recommended adequate preoperative evaluation for every case: Discussion within the group on the operative indication and surgical plan, adequate informed consent with the patient and the family, and to have a national registry for all the cases. Following the recommendation, Japanese Society of Gastroenterological Surgery has started an online registry where all the cases of laparoscopic hepatectomy, except for partial hepatectomy and left lateral sectionectomy, must be registered preoperatively with the intended surgical plan to maintain external evaluation of the surgical indication. Surgical data and complications must be registered once the surgery is completed and the patient is discharged. This type of national registry system maintains the quality of the surgery performed in the country.

LACK OF OVERVIEW

One of the major concerns of laparoscopic surgery compared to open surgery is a lack of overview. While we get magnified views of the several small vessels, it is often easy to lose track of the anatomy. Especially in hepatectomy, losing track of anatomy and deviating from the intended line of resection can result into injuring major vessels or tumor. Several technologies can help the surgeon to keep track of the anatomy during resection. Laparoscopic ultrasound should be routinely performed to check for the location of tumor, major vessels, and their relationship with the intended line of resection. Preoperative simulation with three-dimensional (3D) computed tomography (CT) can help surgeons to understand the anatomy and what to expect in the line of resection **(Fig. 2)**. In recent years, an advancement in fluoroscopy has made it possible to use indocyanine green (ICG) preoperatively to check the location of the tumor during resection or use it after clamping the Glisson to check for the demarcation line.

OUR EXPERIENCE

Steel Memorial Muroran Hospital is a small community-based hospital with around 600 gastrointestinal surgeries every year with nearly 80% of them being laparoscopic surgery. We are a low-volume center and perform roughly 10–15 laparoscopic liver resections every year.

Our approach to laparoscopic hepatectomy has been pure laparoscopic from the beginning. While with hand-assisted methods and hybrid approach can help compensate for the technical aspects of laparoscopic hepatectomy, it loses the benefits of laparoscopic surgery such as reduced blood loss and complications. It is important to become technically proficient in laparoscopic surgery before attempting laparoscopic liver resections. Animal training are highly useful in mastering new techniques and are highly recommended even for the experienced laparoscopic surgeons before they attempt new advanced surgeries.

Cadaver training is another way to get accustomed to the anatomy; however, in liver resection, one of the major concerns is hemostasis, which cannot be replicated in cadaver trainings. As laparoscopic hepatectomy is a team surgery, training with the team is important. Visiting high-volume centers and observing their techniques, management of instruments and complications can also be very educational for the centers looking forward to introducing laparoscopic hepatectomies.

For all liver resections, our preoperative evaluations include contrast CT scans and magnetic resonance imaging (MRI) scans, ultrasonography, blood work up, and liver function is tested using ICG 15 minutes retention test. This is a simple test where the patient is injected with 0.5 mg/kg of ICG into peripheral blood vessel and blood sample taken exactly 15 minutes after the injection from another site is tested for the level of ICG. The result of ICG determines resection limitation of the patients according to the Makuuchi criteria (**Flowchart 1**).[11] We use Synapse Vincent™ software by FUJIFILM to create a 3D image of the liver and its vessels and simulate the plane of

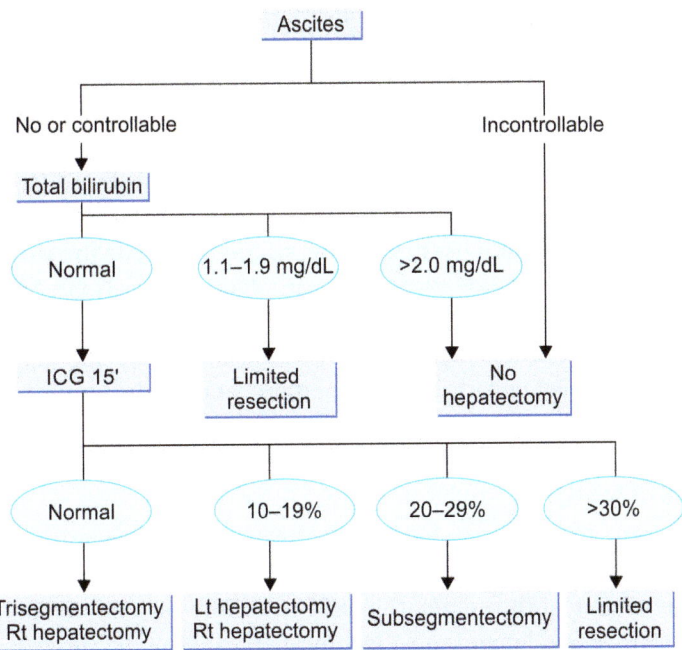

Flowchart 1: Makuuchi criteria for liver resection.[11]

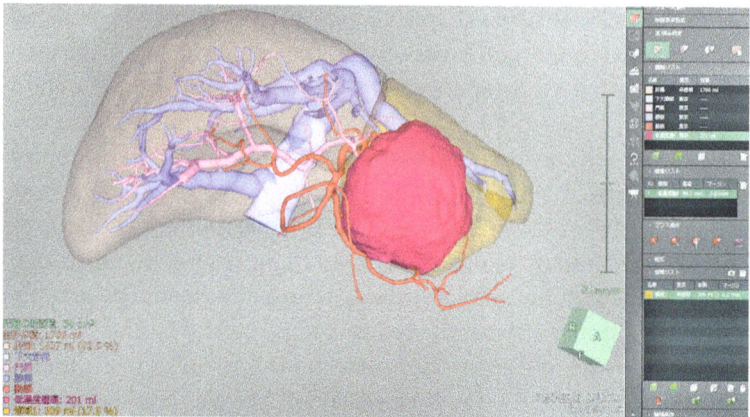

Fig. 2: Three-dimensional (3D) computed tomography (CT) using SYNAPSE Vincent Software™.

resection preoperatively **(Fig. 2)**. This image helps us navigate during the surgery. This software also helps us calculate the liver volume and the expected volume of remaining liver after the resection. We can do simulation with various lines of resections and surgical technique and check for the volume of the remnant liver. This along with the liver function tests helps us determine the best possible surgery for the patient and minimizing the risk of posthepatectomy hepatic failure.

As in open resections, we employ Pringle maneuver in almost all of laparoscopic hepatectomies. Avascular plane of lesser omentum is first divided, then a rubber vessel tape is passed through the Winslow foramen to tape the hepatoduodenal ligament. This tape is pulled out of one of the 5 mm ports and the port is removed. The tape is passed through a rubber tube which is then introduced into to the abdomen. Pulling the vessel tape and pushing the rubber tube is used to clamp the hepatoduodenal ligament **(Fig. 3)**.

For liver resections, we employ the combinations of clamp crush technique using Biclamps® or Ligasure® or using CUSA®. With Biclamps® and CUSA®, the assistant uses Harmonic scalpel® to divide the small vessels and soft coagulation mode for hemostasis. Medium vessels are clipped and divided. Larger vessels such as main branches of Glisson and main hepatic veins are divided using staplers. Navigation using 3D CT and laparoscopic ultrasound is done regularly to check for the location of the tumor and vessels and our line of resection.

■ CONCLUSION

Laparoscopic hepatectomy has many advantages over open hepatectomy. However, before starting with laparoscopic hepatectomy, we need to consider the case volume of the center, the difficulty of the case we are attempting, the experience and laparoscopic technical expertise of the surgeon and the

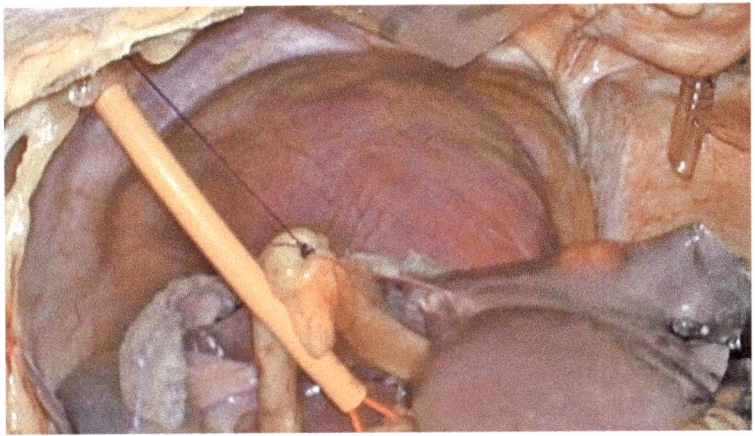

Fig. 3: Pringle maneuver.

surgical team involved in the surgery and the bailout method when things do not work out.

■ REFERENCES

1. Reich H, McGlynn F, DeCaprio J, Budin R. Laparoscopic excision of benign liver lesions. Obstet Gynecol. 1991;78(5 Pt 2):956-8.
2. Azagra JS, Goergen M, Gilbart E, Jacobs D. Laparoscopic anatomical (hepatic) left lateral segmentectomy-technical aspects. Surg Endosc. 1996;10(7):758-61.
3. Kaneko H, Takagi S, Shiba T. Laparoscopic partial hepatectomy and left lateral segmentectomy: technique and results of a clinical series. Surgery. 1996;120(3):468-75.
4. Xu H, Liu F, Li H, Wei Y, Li B. Outcomes following laparoscopic versus open major hepatectomy: a meta-analysis. Scand J Gastroenterol. 2017;52(12):1307-14.
5. Jin B, Chen MT, Fei YT, Du SD, Mao YL. Safety and efficacy for laparoscopic versus open hepatectomy: a meta-analysis. Surg Oncol. 2018;27(2):A26-34.
6. Cipriani F, Ratti F, Cardella A, Catena M, Paganelli M, Aldrighetti L. Laparoscopic versus open major hepatectomy: analysis of clinical outcomes and cost effectiveness in a high-volume center. J Gastrointest Surg. 2019;23(11):2163-73.
7. Ban D, Kudo A, Ito H, Mitsunori Y, Matsumura S, Aihara A, et al. The difficulty of laparoscopic liver resection. Updates Surg. 2015;67(2):123-8.
8. Brown KM, Geller DA. What is the learning curve for laparoscopic major hepatectomy? J Gastrointest Surg. 2016;20(5):1065-71.
9. Hong SK, Suh KS, Yoon KC, Lee JM, Cho JH, Yi NJ, et al. The learning curve in pure laparoscopic donor right hepatectomy: a cumulative sum analysis. Surg Endosc. 2019;33(11):3741-8.
10. Nomi T, Fuks D, Kawaguchi Y, Mal F, Nakajima Y, Gayet B. Learning curve for laparoscopic major hepatectomy. Br J Surg. 2015;102(7):796-804.
11. Makuuchi M, Kosuge T, Takayama T, Yamazaki S, Kakazu T, Miyagawa S, et al. Surgery for small liver cancers. Semin Surg Oncol. 1993;9(4):298-304.

CHAPTER

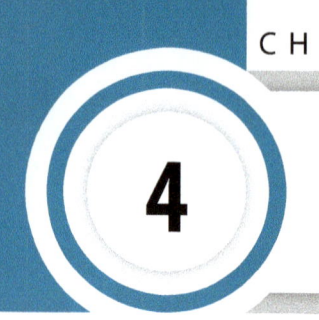

Role of Indocyanine Green in Laparoscopic Liver Surgery

Katherine M Panganiban, Catherine SC Teh

INTRODUCTION

Indocyanine green (ICG) is a water-soluble fluorophore that binds to plasma proteins in the human body, taken up by the hepatocytes and secreted unmetabolized by the bile. It is rapidly cleared in the bloodstream within 5–8 minutes in patients with a healthy liver providing a high margin of safety as a dye for use in fluorescence-guided surgery (FGS).[1] Known contraindications include pregnancy, breastfeeding, and allergy to iodine.

On exposure to near-infrared (NIR) light, at a wavelength of 778–830 nm, the protein-bound dye produces fluorescence on the targeted tissue. Initially used for photography, ICG found its use for liver function testing and angiography of retinal veins in 1957.[2,3] Since then, many clinical applications of this fluorophore dye were discovered. It was in 2009 when Ishizawa et al. noted that ICG has been retained in primary and metastatic liver tumors after preoperative injection.[4] Continued interest and further investigations on clinical applications of fluorescence imaging (FI) using ICG in open, laparoscopic, thoracoscopic, or robotic surgery are noted dynamically, thereafter. It is cost-effective, contributory to surgeon's intraoperative decision real-time, does not change the look of the surgical field, and has a minimal learning curve for users.

BASIC PRINCIPLES IN FLUORESCENCE IMAGING WITH INDOCYANINE GREEN

Fluorescence is produced when proteins in the human bile (albumin and lipoprotein) bind with indocyanine green [injected peripherally via intravenous (IV) route, or directly into the targeted structure] is exposed to NIR light and detected by a specialized camera and scope for fluorescence guided surgery, on a tissue depth of not >10 mm.[4] In hepatobiliary surgery, the usual dose of ICG administered is 0.25–0.5 mg/mL and the timing of administration is dependent on the planned procedure. It has a high detection rate for superficial tumors and for small lesions missed on preoperative and intraoperative ultrasound (IOUS). For deeper tumors, further dissection is needed to be able to eventually appreciate the fluorescence. In our experience, IOUS is done routinely. The combination of FI with other imaging studies increases the detection rate of lesions and possible pathologies.

It optimizes the safety of our patients perioperatively by increasing the surgeon's visualization of structures. Also, it is beneficial in laparoscopic and robotic surgery, where there is limitation in gross inspection of a pathology or visualization of structures, and tactile feedback is lacking.[5]

IMAGING GOAL AND TARGET STRUCTURE

Indocyanine green fluorescence is highly detected in hepatobiliary system due to the fluorophore's biliary excretion and bile-binding capacity. Prior to performance of fluorescence-guided surgery using ICG dye, it is significant to know the imaging goal and target structure. These parameters are important to keep in mind in planning for the ICG dye dosing and timing of administration.

Imaging goal can be any of the following: (1) Anatomical identification, (2) vascular angiography, (3) perfusion assessment, or (4) early detection of a possible complication, such as hypoperfusion on anastomotic site and bile leakage.

OVERVIEW OF CLINICAL APPLICATIONS OF FLUORESCENCE IMAGING USING INDOCYANINE GREEN

Similarly, it is imperative to know what we want to see. For example, is it the common bile duct or the cystic artery? Or is it the pathologic segment of the liver or the surrounding area?

Target structures may be of a normal anatomy, an anatomical variation, or a pathology. It can also be an arterial or a venous supply on vascular angiography. Knowing the presence or abundance of receptors on the cell surface, its subcellular organelle, or the membrane transporter substrate of the target structure are of key concerns, since all FI techniques are dependent on concentration, abundance, and the availability of the target. For example, in areas where biliary stasis is present, such as in cases of liver lesions, the fluorophore can be accumulated within the parenchyma and/or the periphery of the tumor, projected as fluorescence upon exposure to NIR light.

In keeping the imaging goal and target structures in mind, we can plan on the administration of the fluorophore and maximize its use during the surgery.

INDOCYANINE GREEN FLUOROPHORE ADMINISTRATION: DOSAGE AND TIMING

Of equal importance with imaging goal and target structure is the ICG dosage and timing of administration. These are important in optimizing the visualization produced by FI. Also, ICG dosage and timing of administration need to be established in standardization of FI in clinical practice.

With regards to the fluorophore administration, we think that knowledge on the key phases of FI using ICG is important prior to performing FGS. According to Vahrmeijer et al.[6], there are four key phases in FI: (1) Administration, (2) vascular phase, (3) distribution, and (4) post clearance.

Indocyanine green administration may be done through IV injection, directly into the targeted structure, or oral (preparation not available in all countries) administration route. In detail, we will discuss later on this chapter the optimal dosage and timing of administration of the fluorophore per clinical application, focusing on FI in hepatobiliary surgery. The second is the vascular phase 2 (or the accumulation phase 2 via the oral route)—arterial followed by venous phase. Arterial phase is fast and keen observation is needed to appreciate arterial fluorescence. In our experience, this occurs within the first 15-150 seconds upon peripheral IV administration. Coordination with the anesthesiologist or nurse who will administer the dye should be done. Venous fluorescence occurs, thereafter. At this point, the arterial fluorescence will disappear. In our experience, peak of venous fluorescence starts within 3-5 minutes after IV administration. Distribution phase 2 comes next. This phase starts when the fluorophore reaches its half-life. Intraoperatively, distribution phase is taking place when you see that fluorescence becomes apparent in the liver parenchyma. In our experience, this starts at about 10-15 minutes after IV administration. This is also the stage wherein the liver parenchyma is highly fluorescent as compared to the surrounding structures. Also, other highly vascularized organs such as the stomach and the bowel segments will be noted to have fluorescence. The last phase is the post-hepatic clearance phase, occurring >15 minutes to hours after the administration. This phase is continually occurring parallel with tissue biodistribution and target binding. Signal-to-background ratio (SBR) is the fluorescence on the target site (i.e., signal from a liver lesion) in contrast with the background (i.e., liver parenchyma) fluorescence.[7] SBR on the target increases as the fluorophore is cleared from the bloodstream and normal tissues. Knowing the key phases in FI using ICG and the principle behind the SBR is contributory to the adequate dosing and effective timing of ICG administration preoperatively. All of these are contributory to the optimal visualization of the surgical field when performing FGS.

INDOCYANINE GREEN SYSTEMS

Indocyanine green systems improve visualization of surgeons on the field. This addresses the issue of the "visual perception illusion", which according to Osayi et al. is the primary cause of error in 97% of cases in bile duct injuries.[8] In addition to understanding the basic principles of FI, familiarity with different ICG systems is also contributory.

A complete system is composed of an NIR-capable light source, scope, camera, and control switch for FI. Fluorescence activation may be voice-activated, hand-controlled, or foot-controlled. ICG systems are simple and safe to use. They provide intraoperative imaging real-time, without impeding the clinical workflow.

Different ICG systems are available in the market for open, laparoscopic, and robotic surgery. For open surgery: Photodynamic Eye (PDE), Hyper Eye Medical System (HEMS), Fluobeam, Artemis, Solaris, Quest Spectrum, Curadel ResVet LAB-Flare, Visionsense Iridium, SPY-Elite, SPY-fi, and VITOM. For laparoscopic surgery: Olympus Visera, Stryker, Novadaq, Karl Storz Image 1S, and Viron X. For robotic surgery: DaVinci Firefly.

CLINICAL APPLICATIONS IN HEPATOBILIARY SURGERY

Indocyanine green and FI has been widely developed in hepatobiliary surgery achieving clinical applicability from liver function testing to tumor identification, liver segmentation, biliary anatomy, perfusion assessment, and even detection of possible complications. In near future, these FI applications may become standards of practice in hepatobiliary surgery as an adjunct tool for safe surgery.

LIVER TUMOR IDENTIFICATION AND LOCALIZATION

One of the key applications of FI using ICG in hepatobiliary surgery is in tumor identification and localization in the liver. At a standard dose of 0.5 mg/kg for liver surgery, administered intravenously, liver tumors within 8 mm from the liver surface or the cut surface of the liver parenchyma may be identified and localized. Timing of administration varies from 1 to 14 days prior to planned operation based on underlying liver pathology.[9] We administer intravenously the recommended dosage of the dye, there to 5 days prior to scheduled surgery for noncirrhotic livers, and 5-7 days for cirrhotic livers, allowing us optimum visualization of the liver lesion, without the fluorescence on the surrounding normal liver parenchyma.

Upon exposure to NIR-light, different intraoperative fluorescence patterns may be appreciated depending on the pathology and differentiation of the tumor. Ishizawa et al. identified three fluorescence patterns in liver tumors: Total fluorescence, partial fluorescence, and rim fluorescence. Total fluorescence is seen on well-differentiated hepatocellular carcinoma (HCC), and rim or peripheral type of fluorescence is commonly seen on poorly differentiated HCC and colorectal liver metastasis (CRLM).[10] Both primary and secondary liver malignancies can be identified using FI. The characterization of these fluorescence patterns is mainly through biliary excretion disorders present in cancerous tissues of HCC and in noncancerous tissues around the foci of an adenocarcinoma. In another study by Ishizawa et al., immunohistochemical staining and gene expression analysis further explained the mechanism of ICG-fluorescence in HCCs.[11] According to deGraaf, in well-differentiated HCC tumors, expression levels of portal uptake ICG transporters (organic anion-transporting polypeptide 8 and Na$^+$/taurocholate co-transporting polypeptide 9) are well-preserved, but functional or morphological biliary excretion disorders are present, leading to retention of ICG in cancerous tissues.[12] On the other hand, in poorly differentiated HCCs, the portal uptake transporters are downregulated in cancerous tissues but biliary excretion of ICG by surrounding noncancerous hepatic parenchyma is also impaired, resulting in rim or peripheral type of fluorescence. Similarly, in CRLM, the rim-type fluorescence has been reported to be caused by immature hepatocytes with decreased bile excretion ability surrounding the tumor.[13] A study by Shibasaki et al. found that this pattern of ICG fluorescence of HCC tissues is associated with a risk of recurrence after liver surgery.[14]

To date, the role of ICG-FI in cholangiocarcinoma has been described in very few cases.[15, 16] In contrast with some authors,[17] our case showed a hypofluorescent pattern. Indeed, hepatocytes accumulating ICG are usually absent in this tumor; thus, cholangiocarcinoma appears as a hypofluorescent area surrounded by a hyperfluorescent ring. This latter has been attributed to compressed thin biliary ducts containing ICG, with concomitant intrahepatic cholestasis produced by the tumor itself. Interestingly, our case showed a central hypofluorescent area (constituted by neoplastic biliary cells) surrounded by a thin hyperfluorescent ring represented by HCC without areas of cholestasis. To the best of our knowledge, this is the first time that the ICG-FI pattern of a mixed cholangiohepatocarcinoma has been reported. Like cholangiocarcinoma, metastatic liver tumors also appear as hypofluorescent nodules because they do not accumulate ICG.[18] The characteristic hyperfluorescent rim surrounding the tumor is believed to be constituted by compressed hepatocytes, with increased ductular transformation and severe disorders of bile excretion.[19]

Fluorescence imaging has a high sensitivity and detection rate for liver tumor identification and localization due to improved visualization in and around the target lesion. This aids in intraoperative decision-making serving as a guide in liver resection that aids in parenchymal sparing liver resection, and possibly reduce the risk of positive margins.[20,21] In our experience of FI with ICG in 39 liver resections, a 100% identification rate of target lesions was achieved with 87% preoperative imaging studies correlation; 97% correlation with IOUS; and 95% correlation with histopathology margins of resection.[22]

Although FI with ICG has a high detection rate for target lesions, reports of high false-positivity rate up to 40% demand further research regarding the timing, dosage, and interface with the various systems currently available.[23]

The following factors are contributory to false-positive fluorescence of lesions: Cirrhotic liver, dysplastic nodules, <24-hour interval between administration of ICG and operation, bile duct proliferation, necrosis, and presence of other liver lesions such as cysts, hemangioma, and atypical nonmalignant lesions. Incidence of false-positives may be reduced by administering ICG at least 3–7 days prior to surgery, especially in patients with decreased liver function due to cirrhosis or preoperative chemotherapy.[24] Clinical correlation of these false-positive lesions is necessary for intraoperative decision-making.

Surgical resection of primary and metastatic liver tumors is considered as the gold standard in treatment. However, postoperative intrahepatic recurrence rates remain significant, even after potentially curative surgery. The presence of undetected lesions during liver surgery could lead to disease underestimation, particularly for small and subcapsular lesions that are very difficult to detect preoperatively even by current advanced diagnostic imaging. ICG-FI may thus serve as an adjunct in detecting these lesions. Innovations and improvements in detecting these lesions are pivotal to detect intraoperatively and remove all resectable lesions.[25]

Irrespective of their fluorescence patterns, subcapsular hepatic tumors can be identified on the liver surfaces by intraoperative FI, following preoperative IV injection of ICG. In this technique, ICG (0.5 mg/kg body weight) is administered intravenously, usually within 2 weeks before surgery. This method can also be used to detect biliary congestion caused by tumor invasion, micro metastases from pancreatic cancer, and extrahepatic spread of HCC.[26-28] The intraoperative ICG-FI of hepatic tumors is simple and is especially useful for identifying subcapsular lesions during laparoscopic hepatectomy.[29]

In our experience, ICG-FI identified all previously known hepatic lesions and detected further small subcapsular tumors undiagnosed by conventional procedures, with a resulting 20% diagnostic improvement. This finding confirms the utility of ICG-FI for more accurate disease staging.[30] However, in our present and previous experiences, the total sensitivity of ICG-FI still remains fairly limited because lesions at >8 mm of liver depth may escape detection. On the other hand, ICG-FI confers the surgeon the remarkable advantages to guide hepatic resection in a real-time fashion and to immediately evaluate surgical margins as a benchtop system.[31] In addition, previous experiences have already demonstrated that ICG-FI-guided surgery during laparoscopic approach to several hepatic tumors may improve staging, oncologic radicality, and avoid unnecessary laparotomies. Finally, ICG-FI may also contribute to improvements in pathological examination because identification of fluorescent regions before microscopic evaluation would allow focused attention to highly suspicious areas.[32]

From a theoretical point of view, three remarks should be taken into consideration. First, in HCC (which obviously contains hepatocytes), ICG can be captured and retained by malignant cells; moreover, the secretion of ICG may be altered due to architectural disorders reducing the possibility of excretion. Second, if the tumor is formed by nonhepatocellular cells, as in the case of metastases, ICG could be retained by a group of hepatocytes surrounding the nodule and compressed by the nodule itself. Third, if the nodule contains predominantly epithelial cells that are normally part of the biliary ducts (cholangiocarcinoma), they should not absorb the dye and should behave in a manner similar to metastases but with greater alterations in biliary delivery processes.[33]

LIVER SEGMENT VISUALIZATION

Boundaries of hepatic segments can be visualized following injection of 0.25–2.5 mg/mL ICG into the portal veins or by IV injection of 2.5 mg ICG following closure of the proximal portal pedicle toward hepatic regions to be removed. These techniques enable identification of hepatic segments before hepatectomy and during parenchymal transection for anatomic resection. Advances in imaging systems will increase the use of fluorescence imaging as an intraoperative navigation tool that can enhance the safety and accuracy of open and laparoscopic/robotic hepatobiliary surgery.

Aoki first described FI of anatomical liver segments following IOUS guided direct portal injection of ICG by in 2008.[34] This is called as the positive staining technique. This technique was later refined by using a more diluted solution of ICG (2.5 mg) as a source of fluorescence and an imaging system enabling fusion of fluorescence images on color images.[35] A negative staining technique can also be done by intraoperative IV injection of ICG of at least 0.25 mg following closure/division of a hepatic segment portal pedicles. The corresponding occluded segments will not demonstrate any fluorescence, while the nonoccluded liver segments will fluorescence **(Fig. 1)**. This latter technique is especially useful in laparoscopic hepatic segmentectomy, where the positive staining method of direct portal vein injection of ICG is technically more challenging.[36,37]

BILIARY TREE MAPPING

In 2009, fluorescence cholangiography during laparoscopic cholecystectomy was first described.[6] The source of this incisionless cholangiography was the IV injection of ICG at least 15 minutes prior to surgery. The fluorescence in the biliary tree was noted even up to 6 hours after injection. This has the potential advantage over conventional radiographic cholangiography in saving time and avoiding bile duct injury associated with the catheterization required for injection of contrast materials.

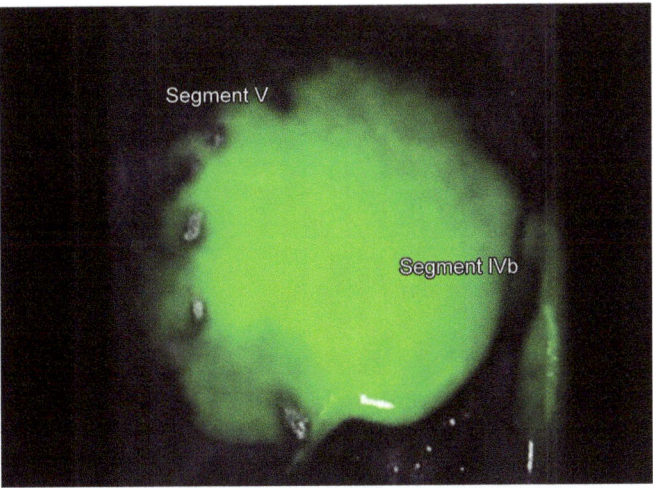

Fig. 1: Negative staining technique for liver segmentation.

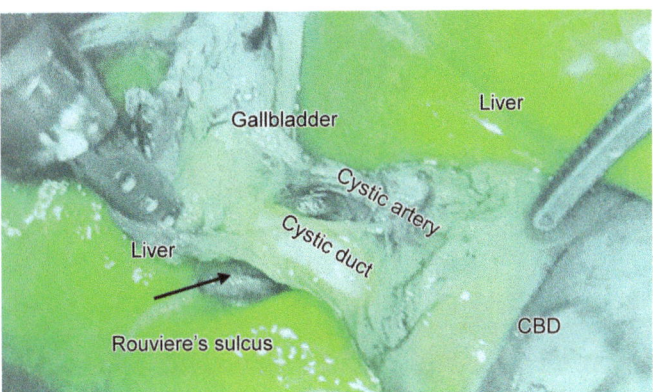

Fig. 2: Incisionless cholangiography.

Although fluorescence cholangiography has a limitation in detecting small stones floating in the common bile duct, the present technique has recently gained attention as a novel and easy-to-use navigation tool that provides a roadmap of the extrahepatic ducts, enhancing safety during laparoscopic[38] and robotic cholecystectomy [39] and reducing the need for intraoperative radiographic cholangiography **(Fig. 2)**.

In a systematic review published in 2017, 19 studies were analyzed. There was moderate-quality evidence that ICG-assisted visualization of the extrahepatic bile duct is superior to intraoperative cholangiogram [relative risk (RR) = 1.16; 95% confidence interval (CI): 1.00–1.35].[40] While the difference was not significant in that study, it was significant in some other single-center series.[41] Considering the relative ease and speed of the procedure, in the future, ICG-based visualization of the biliary anatomy might replace

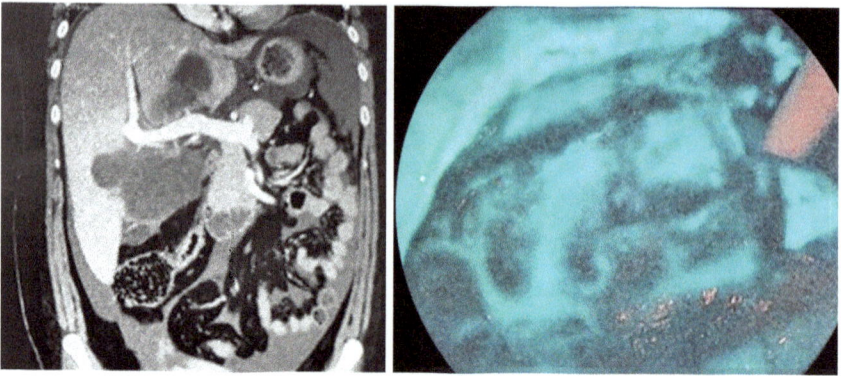

Fig. 3: Intrahepatic biliary anatomy.

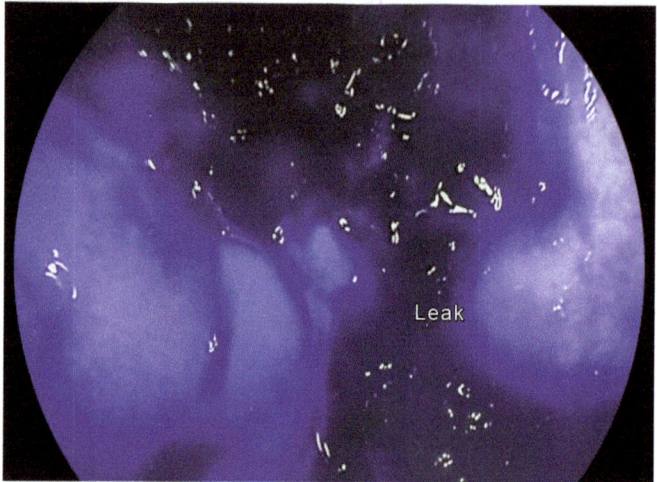

Fig. 4: Post-hepatectomy bile leak.

intraoperative cholangiography, which requires a preliminary dissection of the confluence between the cystic and bile ducts and cannulation of the structures.

With the aim of overcoming the limits of retrospective data, we await the results of a prospective randomized controlled trial (FALCON) comparing INR fluorescence cholangiography-assisted laparoscopic cholecystectomy versus conventional laparoscopic cholecystectomy.[42]

Intrahepatic biliary anatomy can likewise be defined by FI with ICG during liver parenchymal dissection **(Fig. 3)**. Bile leak may also be detected in real time after liver transection is completed **(Fig. 4)**.

This is especially useful to immediately repair or ligate bile ducts intraoperatively to avoid postoperative complications. In our series, three cases of bile leaks were detected and repaired immediately.

REFERENCES

1. Meijer DK, Weert B, Vermeer GA. Pharmacokinetics of biliary excretion in man. VI. Indocyanine green. Eur J Clin Pharmacol. 1988;35(3):295-303.
2. Guyer DR, Puliafito CA, Monés JM, Friedman E, Chang W, Verdooner SR. Digital indocyanine-green angiography in chorioretinal disorders. Ophthalmology. 1992;99:287-91.
3. Reinhart MB, Huntington CR, Blair LJ, Heniford BT, Augenstein VA. Indocyanine green: historical context, current applications, and future considerations. Surg Innov. 2016;23(2):166-75.
4. Nakaseko Y, Ishizawa T, Saiura A. Fluorescence-guided surgery for liver tumors. J Surg Oncol. 2018;118(2):324-31
5. Alander JT, Kaartinen I, Laakso A, Pätilä T, Spillmann T, Tuchin VV, et al. A review of indocyanine green, fluorescent imaging in surgery. Int J Biomed Imaging. 2012;2012:940585.
6. Vahrmeijer A, Hutteman M, van der Vorst J, van de Velde CJH. Image-guided cancer surgery using near-infrared fluorescence. Nat Rev Clin Oncol. 2013;10:507-18.
7. Holt D, Parthasarathy AB, Okusanya O, Keating J, Venegas O, Deshpande C, et al. Intraoperative near-infrared fluorescence imaging and spectroscopy identifies residual tumor cells in wounds. J Biomed Opt. 2015;20(7):76002.
8. Osayi SN, Wendling MR, Drosdeck JM, Chaudhry UI, Perry KA, Noria SF, et al. Near-infrared fluorescent cholangiography facilitates identification of biliary anatomy during laparoscopic cholecystectomy. Surg Endosc. 2015;29:368-75.
9. Galizia G, Auricchio A, Lieto E, Cardella F, Basile N, Castellano P, et al. Indocyanine green fluorescence imaging-guided surgery in primary and metastatic liver tumors. Surg Innov. 2018;25(1):62-8.
10. Ishizawa T, Saiura A, Kokudo N. Clinical application of indocyanine green fluorescence imaging during hepatectomy. Hepato Biliary Surg Nuts. 2015;5(4):322-8.
11. Ishizawa T, Bandai Y, Kokudo N. Fluorescent cholangiography using indocyanine green for laparoscopic cholecystectomy: an initial experience. Arch Surg. 2009;144(4):381-2.
12. de Graaf W, Häusler S, Heger M, van Ginhoven TM, van Cappellen G, Bennink RJ, et al. Transporters involved in the hepatic uptake of (99m) Tc- mebrofenin and indocyanine green. J Hepatol. 2011;54:738-45.
13. Vander Vorst JR, Schaafsma BE, Hutteman M, Verbeek FPR, Liefers GJ, Hartgrink HH, et al. Near-infrared fluorescence-guided resection of colorectal liver metastases. Cancer. 2013;119(18):3411-8.
14. Shibasaki Y, Sakaguchi T, Hiraide T, Morita Y, Suzuki A, Baba S, et al. Expression of indocyanine green-related transporters in hepatocellular carcinoma. J Surg Res. 2015;193(2):567-76.
15. Lieto E, Galizia G, Cardella F, Mabilia A, Basile N, Castellano P, Orditura M, Auricchio A. Indocyanine green fluorescence imaging-guided surgery in primary and metastatic liver tumors. Surg Innov. 2018;25(1):62-68.
16. Miyata A, Ishizawa T, Tani K, Shimizu A, Kaneko J, Aoki T, et al. Reappraisal of a dye-staining technique for anatomic hepatectomy by the concomitant use of indocyanine green fluorescence imaging. J Am Coll Surg. 2015;221(2):e27-36.
17. Ishizawa T, Zuker NB, Kokudo N, Gayet B. Positive and negative staining of hepatic segments by use of fluoresceimaging techniques during laparoscopic hepatectomy. Arch Surg. 2012;147(4):393-4.

18. Ishizawa T, Gumbs AA, Kokudo N, Gayet B. Laparoscopic segmentectomy of the liver: from segment I to VIII. Ann Surg. 2012;256(6):959-64.
19. Inoue Y, Saiura A, Arita J, Yu T. Hepatic vein-oriented liver resection using fusion indocyanine green fluorescence imaging. Ann Surg. 2015;262(6):e98-99.
20. Morita Y, Sakaguchi T, Unno N, Shibasaki Y, Suzuki A, Fukumoto K, et al. Detection of hepatocellular carcinomas with near-infrared fluorescence imaging using indocyanine green: its usefulness and limitation. Int J Clin. 2013;18(2):232-41.
21. Sahani DV, Kalva SP, Tanabe KK, Hayat SM, O'Neill MJ, Halpern EF, et al. Intraoperative US in patients undergoing surgery for liver neoplasms: comparison with MR imaging. Radiology. 2004;232(3):810-4.
22. Panganiban KM, Teh CSC. ICG applications in hepatobiliary system: of fluorescence, frontiers and false positives. HPB. 2018;20(2):S487-8.
23. Ishizawa T, Masuda K, Urano Y, Kawaguchi Y, Satou S, Kaneko J, et al. Mechanistic background and clinical applications of indocyanine green fluorescence imaging of hepatocellular carcinoma. Ann Surg Oncol. 2014;21:440-8
24. Ishizawa T, Fukushima N, Shibahara J, et al. Real-time identification of liver cancers by using Indocyanine green fluorescent imaging. Cancer. 2009; 115:2491-2504.
25. Galizia G, Auricchio A, Lieto E, Cardella F, Mabilia A, Basile N, Castellano P, et al. Indocyanine green fluorescence imaging-guided surgery in primary and metastatic liver tumors. Surgical Innovation. 2018;25(1):62-8.
26. Ishizawa T Harada N, Ishizawa T, Muraoka A, Ijichi M, Kusaka K, Shibasaki M, et al. Fluorescence navigation hepatectomy by visualization of localized cholestasis from bile duct tumor infiltration. J Am Coll Surg. 2010;210(6):e2-6.
27. Yokoyama N, Otani T, Hashidate H, Maeda C, Katada T, Sudo N, et al. Real-time detection of hepatic micro metastases from pancreatic cancer by intraoperative fluorescence imaging: preliminary results of a prospective study. Cancer. 2012;118(11):2813-9.
28. Satou S, Ishizawa T, Kokudo N, Masuda K, Kaneko J, Aoki T, et al. Indocyanine green, fluorescent imaging for detecting extrahepatic metastasis of hepatocellular carcinoma. J Gastroenterol. 2013;48(10):1136-43.
29. Kudo H, Ishizawa T, Tani K, Harada N, Ichida A, Shimizu A, et al. Visualization of subcapsular hepatic malignancy by indocyanine-green fluorescence imaging during laparoscopic hepatectomy. Surg Endosc. 2014;28(8):2504-8.
30. Panganiban KM, Teh CSC. "Lightsabers" fluorescence imaging in laparoscopic liver surgery. Annals of Laparoscopic and Endoscopic Surgery. 2018;3(8).
31. Lim HJ, Chiow AKH, Lee LS, Tan SS, Goh BK, Koh YX, et al. Novel method of intraoperative liver tumour localisation with indocyanine green and near-infrared imaging. Singapore Med J. 2021;62(4):182-189.
32. Masuda K, Urano Y, Kawaguchi Y, Satou S, Kaneko J, et al. Mechanistic background, and clinical applications of indocyanine green fluorescence imaging of hepatocellular carcinoma. Ann Surg Oncol. 2014;21(2):440-8.
33. Baiocchi GL, Diana M, Boni L. Indocyanine green-based fluorescence imaging in visceral and hepatobiliary and pancreatic surgery: state of the art and future directions. World J Gastroenterol. 2018;24(27):2921-30.
34. Aoki T, Yasuda D, Shimizu Y, Odaira M, Niiya T, Kusano T, et al. Image-guided liver mapping using fluorescence navigation system with indocyanine green for anatomical hepatic resection. World J Surg. 2008;32(8):1763-7.

35. Inoue Y, Arita J, Sakamoto T, Ono Y, Takahashi M, Takahashi Y, et al. Anatomical liver resections guided by 3-dimensional parenchymal staining using fusion indocyanine green fluorescence imaging. Ann Surg. 2015;262(1):105-11.
36. Kawaguchi Y, Ishizawa T, Miyata Y, Yamashita S, Masuda K, Satou S, et al. Portal uptake function in veno-occlusive regions evaluated by real-time fluorescent imaging using indocyanine green. J Hepatol. 2013;58(2):247-53.
37. Boni L, David G, Mangani A, Dionigi G, Rausei S, Spampatti S, Cassinotti E, et al. Clinical applications of indocyanine green (ICG) enhanced fluorescence in laparoscopic surgery. Surg Endosc. 2015;29(7):2046-55.
38. Wang X, Teh CSC, Panganiban KM, Ishizawa T, Cavallucci D, Lee SY, et al. Consensus guidelines for the use of fluorescence imaging in hepatobiliary surgery. Ann Surg. 2021;274(1):97-106.
39. Sharma S, Huang R, Hui S, Smith MC, Chung PJ, Schwartzman A, et al. The utilization of fluorescent cholangiography during robotic cholecystectomy at an inner-city academic medical center. J Robot Surg. 2018;12(3):481-5.
40. Vlek SL, van Dam DA, Rubinstein SM, de Lange-de Klerk ESM, Schoonmade LJ, Tuynman JB, et al. Biliary tract visualization using near-infrared imaging with indocyanine green during laparoscopic cholecystectomy: results of a systematic review. Surg Endosc. 2017;31(7):2731-42.
41. Ambe PC, Plambeck J, Fernandez-Jesberg V, Zarras K. The role of indocyanine green fluoroscopy for intraoperative bile duct visualization during laparoscopic cholecystectomy: an observational cohort study in 70 patients. Patient Saf Surg. 2019;13:2.
42. van den Bos, J, Schols, RM, Luyer, MD, van Dam RM, Vahrmeijer AL, Meijerink WJ, et al. Near-infrared fluorescence cholangiography assisted laparoscopic cholecystectomy versus conventional laparoscopic cholecystectomy (FALCON trial): study protocol for a multicentre randomized controlled trial. BMJ Open. 2016;6(8):e011668.

CHAPTER 5

Laparoscopic Right Hepatectomy

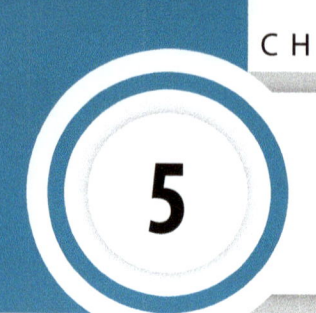

Fumiaki Tokito, Yusuke Ome, Goro Honda, Masakazu Yamamoto

■ INTRODUCTION

We have gradually standardized the various procedures in laparoscopic hepatectomy, finding several advantages of the laparoscopic approach obtained from using a unique laparoscopic caudodorsal view. Among them, the caudate lobe-first approach is remarkably beneficial for laparoscopic right hemihepatectomy (Lap-RH).[1,2]

■ ANATOMY

Anatomically, the origins of the Glissonean branches and hepatic veins are located on the dorsal side of the liver, and they branch similar to a tree, extending toward the ventral side. The hepatic vein trunk runs in the intersegmental plane, which is the border between the sectors, and, theoretically, no Glissonean branch runs in that plane.[3] During anatomical sectionectomy or hemihepatectomy, initiating parenchymal division at the root of the Glissonean tree (i.e., the hepatic hilum) and continuing it toward the periphery with the vertical movement of the instrument make dissection along the intersegmental plane easier. Meanwhile, split injury at the confluences of the hepatic vein branches, which cause severe bleeding, can be prevented by exposing the hepatic vein trunk from the root side toward the periphery.[4,5] Here, we present our standardized procedure of Lap-RH using the caudate lobe-first approach.

■ SURGICAL TECHNIQUE

The patient is placed in the supine position, with only the upper body twisted to the left **(Fig. 1)**. A trocar for the scope is placed at the umbilicus, and the other four trocars are placed beneath the right costal arch **(Fig. 2)**.

Infusion is restricted as much as possible. Pneumoperitoneum is established at 10 mm Hg. Ventilation pressure is maintained as usual.[6] A tourniquet system to Pringle maneuver is prepared through the left hypochondrium, and the Pringle maneuver is initiated when the field cannot be kept dry.[7] To divide the liver parenchyma, we mainly use the CUSA EXcel® system (Integra LifeSciences Corporation, Plainsboro, NJ, USA) with thermal coagulation using the low-voltage electrical cautery mode at the tip of the CUSA EXcel®.

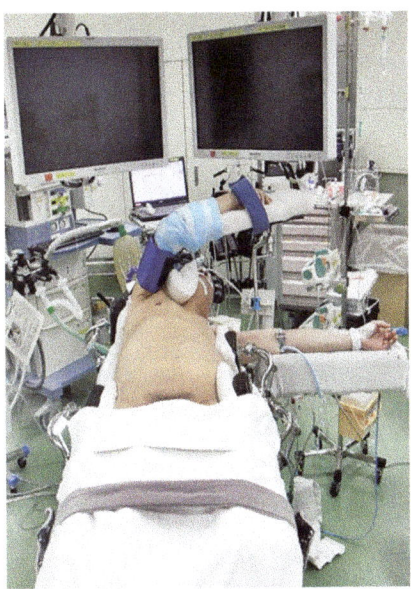

Fig. 1: Patient position. The patient is placed in the supine position, with only the upper body twisted to the left.

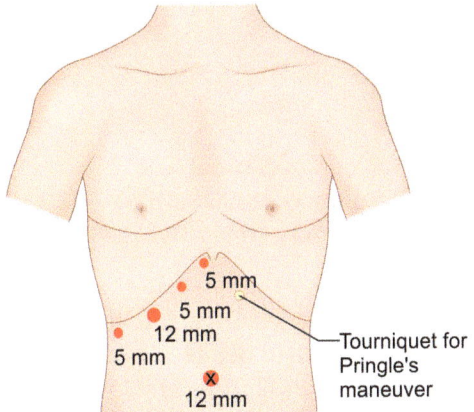

Fig. 2: Trocar placement. A trocar for the scope is placed at the umbilicus, and the other four trocars for the instruments are placed beneath the right costal arch. A tourniquet system for the Pringle maneuver is prepared through the left hypochondrium (green catheter).

The right lobe is usually mobilized before initiating liver dissection. The caudate lobe is detached from the inferior vena cava (IVC) in the unique laparoscopic caudodorsal magnified view, transecting the short hepatic veins. The caudate lobe is cut at the midline from the caudal side parallel to the ventral center line of the IVC (**Fig. 3**). We named this unique approach the caudate lobe-first approach. The caudate lobe is divided at its midline

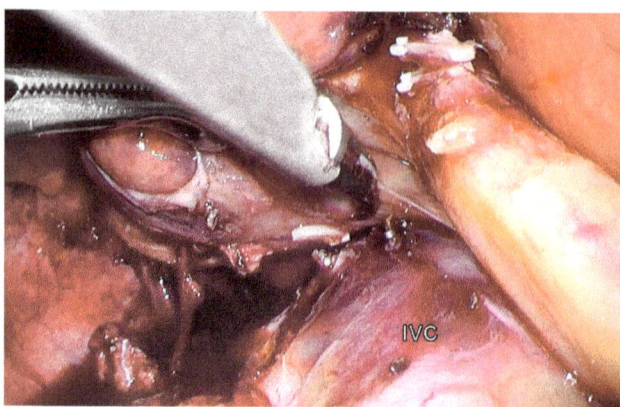

Fig. 3: Caudate lobe-first approach. The caudate lobe is cut at the midline from the caudal side parallel to the ventral center line of the IVC.

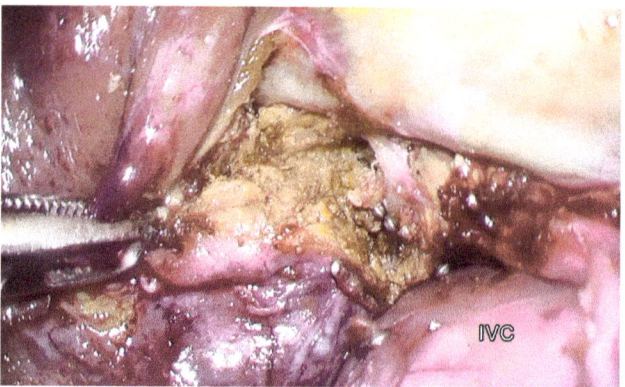

Fig. 4: Dorsal aspect of the right main Glissonean trunk exposed by the caudate lobe-first approach.

from the back parallel with the ventral center line of the IVC. The dorsal aspect of the right main Glissonean trunk is then exposed **(Fig. 4)**. The anterior and posterior Glissonean pedicles are isolated and ligated easily after cholecystectomy because its half dorsal side has already been exposed.

At the cranioventral side of the hilar plate, the liver parenchyma is divided along the major hepatic fissure, which is identified as a demarcation line caused by ligating the right Glissonean pedicles. The root of the drainage vein of segment 5, which often runs closely behind the hepatic hilum, is exposed near the hepatic hilum and divided. The dorsal to the right aspect of the middle hepatic vein (MHV) trunk is exposed continuously toward the IVC side. The cutting plane on the ventral side joined the dorsal cutting plane, which has been previously made by the caudate lobe-first approach. After creating a wide space around the hepatic hilum, the anterior and posterior Glissonean pedicles are separately divided using linear staplers inserted directing from the ventral side to the back side. Linear staplers can be

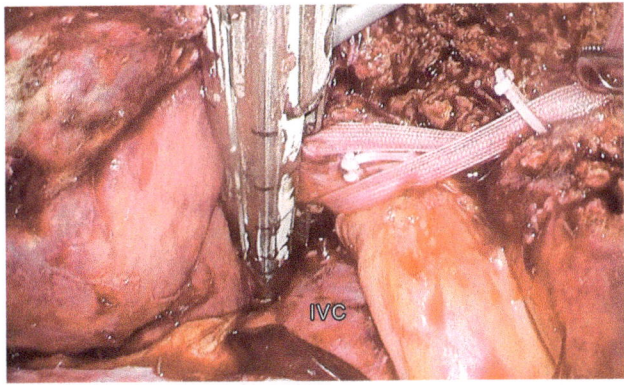

Fig. 5: Division of the Glissonean pedicles. After creating a wide space around the hepatic hilum, the anterior and posterior Glissonean pedicles are separately divided using linear staplers inserted directing from the ventral side to the back side. The posterior Glissonean pedicle is being divided in this picture.

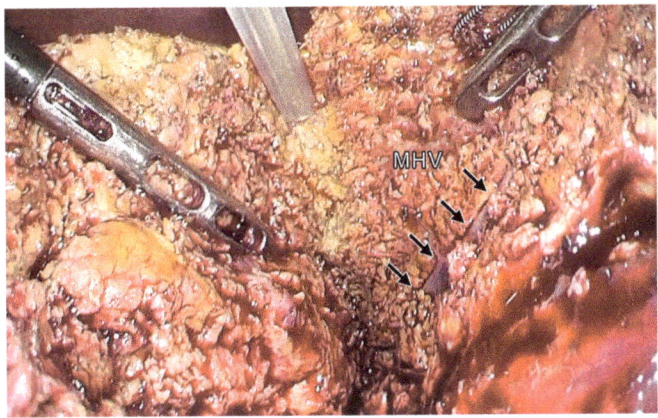

Fig. 6: Middle hepatic vein exposed on the cutting plane of the remnant liver.

inserted safely, because there is a large space that has been prepared behind the Glissonean pedicles by the caudate lobe-first approach **(Fig. 5)**.

The MHV is exposed on the cutting plane of the liver remnant **(Fig. 6)**. Then, parenchymal dissection is advanced between the demarcation line on the liver surface and MHV. In this step, by moving the tip of the CUSA EXcel® from the dorsal toward the ventral side, the parenchymal dissection along the intersegmental plane can be advanced and split injury to the hepatic vein can be avoided. Afterward, division proceeds toward the crotch between the roots of the MHV and right hepatic vein (RHV). After accomplishing parenchymal dissection, the RHV is divided **(Fig. 7)**.

The resected right lobe is enclosed in a plastic bag and removed through the incision in the lower abdomen. A closed suction drain is placed at the right subphrenic space.

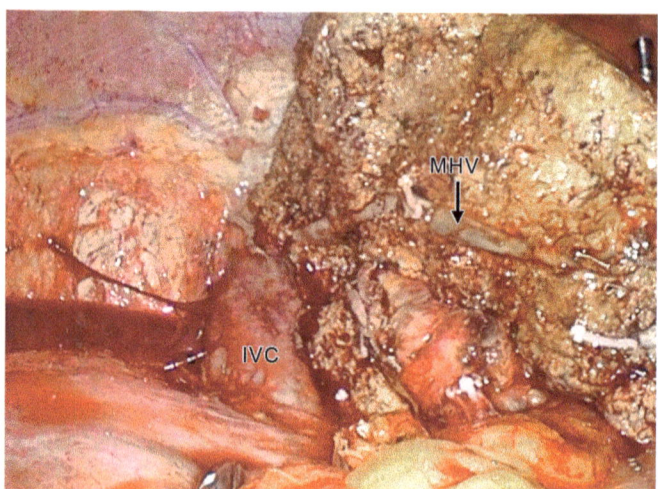

Fig. 7: Final view after completion of right hemihepatectomy.

CONCLUSION

Our standardized procedure of Lap-RH using the caudate lobe-first approach is not only feasible but also confers a true advantage of the laparoscopic approach.

REFERENCES

1. Maeda K, Honda G, Kurata M, Homma Y, Doi M, Yamamoto J, et al. Pure laparoscopic right hemihepatectomy using the caudodorsal side approach (with videos). J Hepatobiliary Pancreat Sci. 2018;25(7):335-41.
2. Homma Y, Honda G, Kurata M, Ome Y, Doi M, Yamamoto J. Pure laparoscopic right posterior sectionectomy using the caudate lobe-first approach. Surg Endosc. 2019;33(11):3851-7..
3. Honda G, Ome Y, Yoshida N, Kawamoto Y. How to dissect the liver parenchyma. Excavation with cavitron ultrasonic surgical aspirator. J Hepatobiliary Pancreat Sci. 2020;27(11):907-12.
4. Honda G, Kurata M, Okuda Y, Kobayashi S, Sakamoto K. Totally laparoscopic anatomical hepatectomy exposing the major hepatic veins from the root side: a case of the right anterior sectorectomy (with video). J Gastrointest Surg. 2014;18(7):1379-80.
5. Honda G, Kurata M, Okuda Y, Kobayashi S, Tadano S, Yamaguchi T, et al. Totally laparoscopic hepatectomy exposing the major vessels. J Hepatobiliary Pancreat Sci. 2013;20(4):435-40.
6. Kobayashi S, Honda G, Kurata M, Okuda Y, Sakamoto K, Tadano S, et al. An experimental study on the relationship among airway pressure, pneumoperitoneum pressure, and central venous pressure in pure laparoscopic hepatectomy. Ann Surg. 2016;263(5):1159-63.
7. Okuda Y, Honda G, Kurata M, Kobayashi S. A useful and convenient procedure for intermittent vascular occlusion in laparoscopic hepatectomy. Asian J Endosc Surg. 2013;6(2):100-3.

CHAPTER

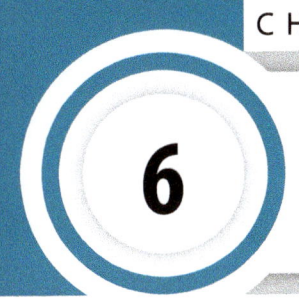

6

Minimal Invasive Treatment for Colorectal Liver Metastases

Giovanni M Garbarino, Giammauro Berardi

■ INTRODUCTION

Despite the progress reached in the multidisciplinary management of colorectal cancer, it still represents a major health issue affecting nearly 1 million people worldwide; moreover, around two-thirds of patients with colorectal cancer develop metastases the liver being the most common site. The treatment of colorectal liver metastasis (CRLM) is based on a multimodal approach including systemic therapies and surgical resection;[1] when these are deemed resectable, surgical approach in combination with chemotherapy represents the standard of care as it offers long-term survival, with rates of 22–55% at 5 years from resection.[2]

Minimally invasive procedures have deeply changed the surgical practice worldwide and have gained interest in the last decades thanks to the improved short-term outcomes such as postoperative complications, hospitalization, esthetics, and overall cost-effectiveness compared to open surgery.[3] The application of minimally invasive techniques to the hepatobiliary field was slower compared to other surgical specialties.[4-8] This was more likely due to the technical difficulties requiring experience in both hepatobiliary and complex laparoscopy, together with a specific long and demanding learning curve.[9,10]

Since the first laparoscopic partial liver resection reported in 1991,[11] the number of laparoscopic liver resections (LLRs) increased constantly, leading to >9,000 LLR reported by Ciria et al. in 2016.[12] From the first Consensus Conference in Louisville and to the recommendations from the Second World Consensus Conference in Morioka, the indications for LLR have been expanded.[12-17] Concerning type of procedures, according to the available evidence, laparoscopy is widely recognized as the gold standard approach for left lateral sectionectomy and for partial resections in the anterolateral segments.[18] Conversely, posterosuperior resections, anatomical segmentectomies, major hepatectomies, central hepatectomy, and right anterior and posterior sectionectomies are certainly more demanding and should be approached after appropriate learning curve.[10] Indeed, various difficulty scoring systems have been formulated to grade the complexity of LLR[19-23] and externally validated in several studies.[24-27] This would allow surgeons embarking on LLR to select and perform procedures appropriate for their level of experience. During the recent Southampton Consensus Guidelines Meeting, LLR for

CRLMs was recommended as a valid alternative to the open approach with shorter hospital stay and lower complication rates;[28] advanced age and obesity were not considered as contraindications while repeated hepatectomies, two-stage resections, proximity to major vessels and lesions >10 cm were considered only in experienced hands as were major hepatectomies, difficult resections (i.e., posterosuperior segments) and anatomical segmentectomies.

Therefore, selection of candidates for LLR should consider patients characteristics, disease presentation, and expertise in order to minimize conversions and to improve postoperative outcomes maintaining safe survivals.[29]

To date, eight meta-analysis pooling studies evaluating the results of >4,000 patients reported comparable oncological outcomes between LLR and open liver resection (OLR) in terms of surgical margins, recurrence rates, overall survival (OS), and disease-free survival (DFS).[30-38] Recently, the long-awaited survival outcomes of the first randomized control trial, the OSLO-COMET, were revealed: median OS was 80 months [95% confidence interval (CI): 52-108] in the LLR group and 81 months (95% CI: 42-120) in the open surgery group ($p = 0.91$).[39]

In 2001, Giulianotti performed the first robotic liver surgery in Italy.[40] Since then, robotic liver resection (RLR) has been slowly adopted as it is believed to overcome some of the limitations of laparoscopy, allowing image-guided surgery from a computerized console.[41] This is very attractive in hepatic surgery due to its complexity, especially in resecting lesions in the posterior-superior segments (VII and VIII). Tumors in these locations require curved transections, which are very challenging with laparoscopy while the robotic arms can overcome these difficulties.[42,43] Nonetheless, the perioperative outcomes of robotic and laparoscopic resections of the posterosuperior segments appear to be similar in terms of blood loss, hospital stay, morbidity, and completeness of resection.[44] Despite the technical advantages, RLR has still a longer operative time and higher costs compared to LLR but comparable blood loss, length of stay, resection margins, and morbidity.[45,46] For those reasons, the robotic approach has been indicated as one treatment option for liver resections with a strong evidence level from the Southampton Consensus Guidelines. However, the recommendation concluded that it can require two trained surgeons to perform procedures and cost-effectiveness studies are mandatory.[28]

LAPAROSCOPIC MINOR LIVER RESECTIONS FOR COLORECTAL LIVER METASTASES

Parenchyma sparing liver resections represent a milestone in the multimodal treatment of CRLM regardless of surgical approach. In fact, compared to more extensive resections, it is associated with less surgical stress and fewer

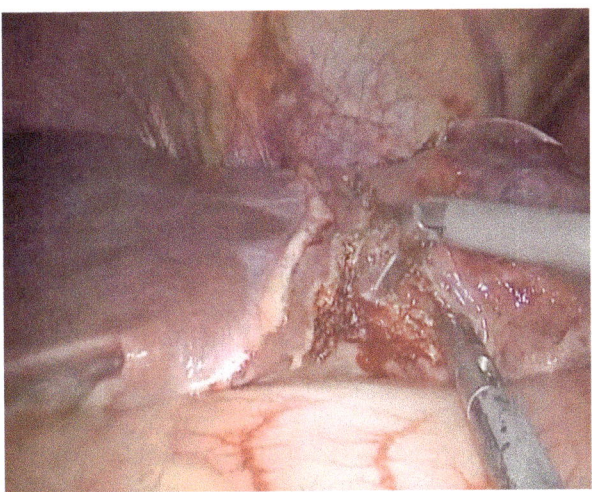

Fig. 1: Laparoscopic left lateral sectionectomy.

complications, especially lower rates of posthepatectomy liver failure that is crucial after neoadjuvant chemotherapy. Moreover, considering the rate of recurrence after resection for CRLM, repeated parenchyma sparing hepatectomies are often necessary and they have been reported to achieve satisfactory outcomes.[47] In this setting, multiple partial nonanatomical resections are performed in order to achieve complete removal of the tumor sparing as much healthy liver as possible **(Fig. 1)**.

Laparoscopic approach for parenchyma sparing resections has been described as safe, with good short- and long-term outcomes. Recently the first randomized control trial, the OSLO-COMET trial, disclosed its results achieving the highest level of evidence currently available on the topic.[39,48] The enrolment of patients was limited to minor LLR for CRLM focusing on mortality, morbidity, and resection margins as principal outcomes: Mortality was comparable between groups, while morbidity was significantly lower in laparoscopy (31% in OLR and 19% in LLR $p = 0.02$). Hospital stay was shorter after LLR and patients required less morphine-based analgesia. Resection margins were comparable between groups with 6% R1 resection rate in LLR and 7% in OLR. Median OS was 80 months (95% CI: 52–108) in the LLR group and 81 months (95% CI: 42–120) in the open surgery group ($p = 0.91$). The results from the OSLO-COMET trial confirm and further enhance the improved postoperative short-term outcomes of LLR compared to OLR without any difference in long-term survivals.

Despite this, the number and the unfavorable localization of multiple tumors could represent a major challenge in laparoscopy due to the need of reaching two different operative fields (right and left liver lobe) in bilobar lesions changing the patient position and the port placement.[49] Furthermore, proficiency in the use of the laparoscopic ultrasound probe is mandatory to locate the lesions and guide the resections in order to achieve safe margins. Nonetheless, Aghayan et al. reported 5-years survival of 44% in 80 patients undergoing laparoscopic parenchymal sparing resections for multiple CRLM.[50]

Overall, the available results demonstrate that laparoscopic parenchyma sparing resections are feasible and represent the preferred option over major resections, because associated with lower postoperative morbidity; more studies are necessary to investigate the role of laparoscopic parenchyma sparing for multiple and bilobar CRLMs as the evidence is still scarce.

LAPAROSCOPIC MAJOR HEPATECTOMIES FOR COLORECTAL LIVER METASTASES

The largest meta-analysis to date has shown that laparoscopic major hepatectomies (LMHs) have less blood loss, morbidity, and length of stay with similar operative times, transfusion rates, and completeness of resection compared to OLR.[12] The Southampton Guidelines stated that the feasibility, reproducibility, and implementation of left and right hepatectomies are sufficiently different that they should be considered separately. Hence, it was advised that their uptake occur at different points in the learning curve.[28,51,52] The percentages of left and right hepatectomies in the LMH case series range between 0 and 55% demonstrating wide variability depending on centers and expertise.[32] In experienced hands, laparoscopic right hemi-hepatectomies are associated with reduced hospital stay and blood loss. Mortality and completeness of resection are comparable to an open approach.[53-55] Laparoscopic left hemihepatectomies have been limited to tertiary referral centers and to experienced surgeons due to the associated technical demands. Compared to an open approach, a laparoscopic approach is associated with reduced blood loss, morbidity, and hospital stay with comparable operative times, completeness of resection, and mortality.[3,32,56-58]

Regarding inflow control and parenchymal transection **(Figs. 2 to 4)**, the guidelines state that the choice of technique is dependent on the characteristics of the disease and the surgeon's preference. Pringle maneuver and the management of intravascular volume to provide a low central venous pressure (CVP) are both essential to reduce blood loss during transection. And, as in open liver surgery, the need for intraoperative ultrasound was considered essential.[28]

In a recent meta-analysis by Kasai et al., LMHs were associated with conversion rates ranging from 9 to 42%.[57] These rates are clearly higher than the average for minor hepatectomies and reasonably reveal the technical difficulty of these procedures. The liver mobilization, the large parenchymal transection surface, and the numbers of potential intraoperative pitfalls certainly represent a major challenge in this setting. Indeed, LMHs should be performed in the final phases of the learning curve, after proficiency is

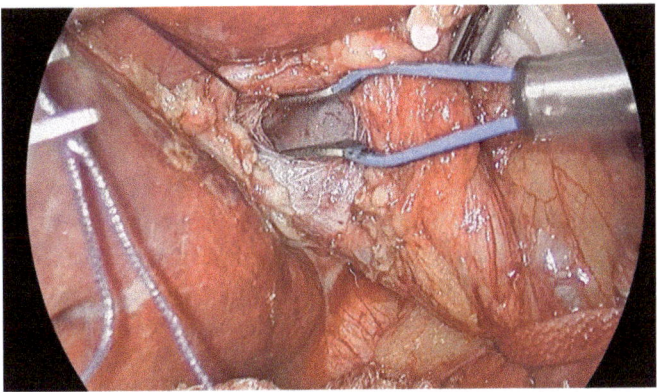
Fig. 2: Dissection of right portal vein for pedicle control.

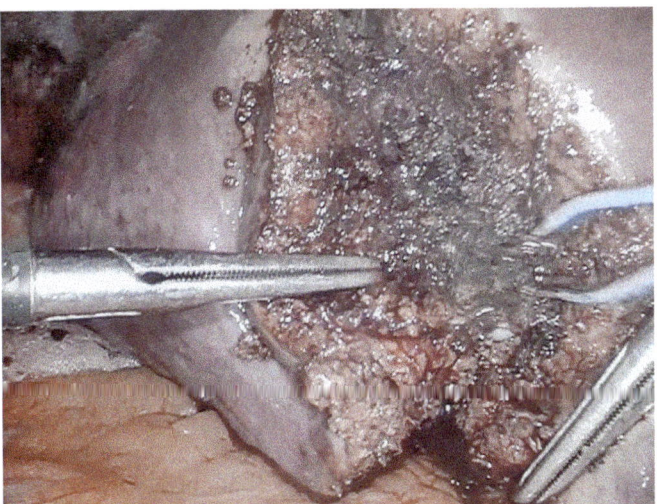
Fig. 3: Right posterior segmentectomy. Use of bipolar for hemostasis.

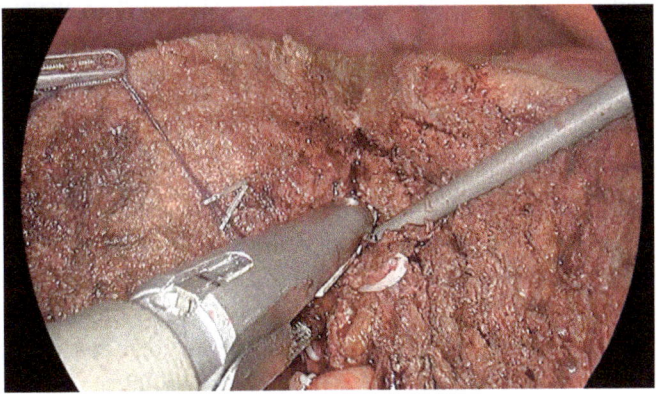
Fig. 4: Use of vascular stapler for portal vein resection.

achieved with minor and easier resections, in order to guarantee safety and improve postoperative outcomes.[52]

To date, only few studies have reported outcomes after laparoscopic extended major hepatectomy (LEMH).[59,60] The potential risks of LEMH compared to standard LMH include a longer operating time, greater intraoperative blood loss, and a higher risk of biliary and vascular complications. Recently Pietrasz et al. compared the perioperative characteristics and postoperative outcomes of LEMH to standard LMH, including 130 (66.7%) patients with CRLM. Despite no differences in postoperative mortality and liver failure, blood loss (400 vs. 214 mL; $p = 0.006$) and overall morbidity (60% vs. 41.5%, $p = 0.052$) were higher in LEMH group. Patients treated with left LEMH experienced more biliary leakage ($p = 0.011$) and more major pulmonary complications ($p = 0.015$) than left LMH. The authors concluded that LEMH is feasible in high-volume centers with experienced surgeons, at the price of important morbidity, with manageable and acceptable outcomes.[61]

The current scientific evidence on LMH, including meta-analysis, suffers from several biases such as the surgeon's experience and the selection of the easier cases for the laparoscopic approach. The results of the first randomized controlled trial (RCT), the ORANGE-II plus (NCT01441856), comparing laparoscopic versus open major hepatectomies, will finally disclose the advantages of one or the other technique in terms of postoperative short- and long-term outcomes.

LAPAROSCOPIC RESECTION OF POSTEROSUPERIOR COLORECTAL LIVER METASTASES

Laparoscopic liver resection of lesions in the posterosuperior segments (PSS) (segments 4a, 7, and 8) are technically very challenging. Indeed the Morioka consensus conference accentuated that laparoscopic resections in these segments must be considered as technically major resections.[14] Experience in both open and laparoscopic surgery is essential to ensure success without compromising the surgical safety and the oncologic efficiency. Therefore, that resections of lesions in the PSS should only be performed by experienced surgeons in high-volume centers.[10,19,28,62]

Several recent reports revealed that patients treated for lesions in PSS benefit the most from a laparoscopic approach, in terms of postoperative outcomes.[63-66] A recent meta-analysis, comparing laparoscopic versus open liver resection for lesions located in the PSS, showed lower overall complication rate (OR 0.50; 95% CI 0.36- 0.70; $p < 0.001$) and postoperative hospital stay (SMD—0.45; 95% CI 0.59–0.30; $p = 0.003$) for patients treated by laparoscopic approach. Concerning the oncological outcomes, no significant difference in R0 resection rate (OR 1.04; 95% CI 0.55–1.96; $p = 0.902$) and DFS for CRLMs (HR 1.05; 95% CI 0.61–1.81) were noted between the groups.[67]

Performing an open resection of a lesion in PSS requires a large incision for its access and exposure resulting in a longer hospital stay and increased morbidity. As reported by Del Pino et al., a significative higher rate of pulmonary complications in patients undergoing OLR for PSS tumors was observed.[68] The access to these deep segments using an open approach can lead to subdiaphragmatic fluid collections and pleural effusion. Moreover, the painful postoperative limitation of the ribcage excursion leads to respiratory dysfunction which increases the risk of pulmonary complications in these patients.

Recently Cipriani et al. demonstrated that laparoscopic approach appears more advantageous for posterosuperior than for anterolateral resections in terms of blood loss and transfusion, morbidity as well as time to functional recovery.[69] Indeed, location of lesions in the PSS has been highlighted as a significant factor to increase difficulty of resections in a number of prediction scores developed for laparoscopic liver resections.[19-21]

Finally, the estimated learning curve of LLR for lesions in the PSS has been reported to be around 40 procedures for wedge resections and 65 surgeries for anatomical resections, being accurate patient selection the key to success.[10]

LAPAROSCOPIC REPEATED LIVER RESECTIONS FOR RECURRENT COLORECTAL METASTASES

Tumor recurrence of CRLMs occurs at a constant rate ranging from 50 to 80% during follow-up after liver resection and in these cases repeat hepatectomy has been shown to provide good oncological outcomes.[47,70-76] Several reports have demonstrated the benefits of a third hepatectomy for patients with recurrent CRLM;[71,72,77] recently a worldwide survey demonstrated the long-term survival benefits up to four repeated liver resections.[71] However, due to the adhesions, the anatomical changes and the hypertrophied liver remnant resulting from previous resections and the chemotherapy-induced liver injury, the rate of intraoperative conversions during laparoscopic repeated hepatectomy may significantly increase.[21] Despite this, some authors reported encouraging results from their experience with laparoscopy for recurrent CRLM.[78,79] In a recent multicenter propensity score matching analysis, LLR was associated with shorter operative time (200 minutes vs. 256 minutes, $p < 0.001$) and shorter hospital stay (5 days vs. 6 days, $p = 0.02$); furthermore, a trend toward less blood loss was noted (200 mL vs. 300 mL, $p = 0.07$), while postoperative morbidity and mortality were comparable between groups. However, these results could have been influenced by the higher rate of primary LLR in the laparoscopic repeated hepatectomy group.[79] Indeed, LLR is generally associated with less postoperative adhesions which could improve accessibility to the abdomen in case of repeated abdominal procedures.

Laparoscopic repeated liver resections are still challenging procedures and should be approached in the late phase of the learning curve by experienced surgeons.

ROBOTIC RESECTIONS FOR COLORECTAL LIVER METASTASES

Over the last two decades, robotic surgery has emerged as a potentially valid alternative to conventional laparoscopic surgery until being validated with a strong evidence level by the Southampton Consensus Guidelines as one treatment option for liver resections.[28]

In fact, a recent systematic review and meta-analysis comparing RLR and LLR suggest that both techniques can be used safely. RLR had significantly longer operating time than LLR (mean: 281 vs. 221 minutes, $p < 0.001$), less blood loss (286 vs. 301 mL, $p < 0.001$), and lower readmission rates [4 vs. 11%, odds ratio (OR): 0.43, CI 95%: 0.24–0.78, $p = 0.005$]. Both techniques appear equivalent in terms of overall and major complications, length of stay, and 30-day and 90-day mortality.[80]

It has been largely described how robotic surgery represents an enhancement of laparoscopy thanks to tremor filtration, three-dimensional stable view, and endowrist instruments, but it still does not overcome some limitations of minimally invasive techniques proficiency gaining.[41,43] These advantages are very attractive in hepatic surgery, especially for the resections of the posterior-superior segments. Tumors in these locations represent a surgical challenge due to convex surface of the liver, the difficulty to achieve an appropriate exposure, and, therefore, the increased risk of bleeding and bile leakage. In this setting, achieving curved transections, suturing, and reaching deep spaces with laparoscopy is very challenging, while the robotic arms can overcome these difficulties.[42,43] Nevertheless, even if the perioperative outcomes of robotic and laparoscopic resections of the posterosuperior segments appear to be similar in terms of blood loss, hospital stay, morbidity, and completeness of resection, the RLR has still a longer operative time and higher costs compared to LLR.[44-46]

In conclusion, an RCT comparing laparoscopic versus robotic liver resections is still lacking and will enable us to draw meaningful conclusions regarding the best minimally invasive approach.

CONCLUSION

Minimally invasive liver resections represent a valid option for the treatment of CRLMs. In several settings, both laparoscopic and robotic liver resections have demonstrated better postoperative outcomes and similar long-term outcomes compared to open resections. The selection of patients, together with the surgeon's experience, still play a crucial role for a successful treatment. Difficult procedures such as major hepatectomies, posterosuperior resections, and recurrent metastases should be referred to high-volume centers with experienced surgeons.

REFERENCES

1. Sugihara K, Uetake H. Therapeutic strategies for hepatic metastasis of colorectal cancer: overview. J Hepatobiliary Pancreat Sci. 2012;19(5):523-7.
2. Simmonds PC, Primrose JN, Colquitt JL, Garden OJ, Poston GJ, Rees M. Surgical resection of hepatic metastases from colorectal cancer: a systematic review of published studies. Br J Cancer. 2006;94(7):982-99.
3. Berardi G, Van Cleven S, Fretland ÅA, Barkhatov L, Halls M, Cipriani F, et al. Evolution of laparoscopic liver surgery from innovation to implementation to mastery: perioperative and oncologic outcomes of 2,238 patients from 4 European specialized centers. J Am Coll Surg. 2017;225(5):639-49.
4. Ghezzi F, Cromi A, Ditto A, Vizza E, Malzoni M, Raspagliesi F, et al. Laparoscopic versus open radical hysterectomy for stage IB2-IIB cervical cancer in the setting of neoadjuvant chemotherapy: a multi-institutional cohort study. Ann Surg Oncol. 2013;20(6):2007-15.
5. Guillou PJ, Quirke P, Thorpe H, Walker J, Jayne DG, Smith AMH, et al. Short-term endpoints of conventional versus laparoscopic-assisted surgery in patients with colorectal cancer (MRC CLASICC trial): multicentre, randomised controlled trial. Lancet. 2005;365(9472):1718-26.
6. Luketich JD, Pennathur A, Awais O, Levy RM, Keeley S, Shende M, et al. Outcomes after minimally invasive esophagectomy: review of over 1000 patients. Ann Surg. 2012;256(1):95-103.
7. Trabulsi EJ, Guillonneau B. Laparoscopic radical prostatectomy. J Urol. 2005; 1(4):196-201.
8. Kitano S, Shiraishi N, Uyama I, Sugihara K, Tanigawa N, Inomata M, et al. A multicenter study on oncologic outcome of laparoscopic gastrectomy for early cancer in Japan. Ann Surg. 2007;245(1):68-72.
9. Gagner M, Rogula T, Selzer D. Laparoscopic liver resection: benefits and controversies. Surg Clin North Am. 2004;84(2):451-62.
10. Berardi G, Aghayan D, Fretland A, Elberm H, Cipriani F, Spagnoli A, et al. Multicentre analysis of the learning curve for laparoscopic liver resection of the posterosuperior segments. Br J Surg. 2019;106(11):1512-22.
11. Reich H, McGlynn F, DeCaprio J, Budin R. Laparoscopic excision of benign liver lesions. Obstet Gynecol. 1991;78(5 Pt 2):956-8.
12. Ciria R, Cherqui D, Geller DA, Briceno J, Wakabayashi G. Comparative short-term benefits of laparoscopic liver resection: 9000 cases and climbing. Ann Surg. 2016;263(4):761-77.
13. Buell JF, Cherqui D, Geller DA, O'Rourke N, Iannitti D, Dagher I, et al. The international position on laparoscopic liver surgery: the Louisville Statement, 2008. Ann Surg. 2009;250(5):825-30.
14. Wakabayashi G, Cherqui D, Geller DA, Buell JF, Kaneko H, Han HS, et al. Recommendations for laparoscopic liver resection: a report from the second international consensus conference held in Morioka. Ann Surg. 2015;261(4):619-29.

15. Cherqui D, Husson E, Hammoud R, Malassagne B, Stéphan F, Bensaid S, et al. Laparoscopic liver resections: a feasibility study in 30 patients. Ann Surg. 2000;232(6):753-62.
16. Descottes B, Lachachi F, Sodji M, Valleix D, Durand-Fontanier S, Pech De Laclause B, et al. Early experience with laparoscopic approach for solid liver tumors: initial 16 cases. Ann Surg. 2000;232(5):641-5.
17. Nguyen KT, Gamblin TC, Geller DA. World review of laparoscopic liver resection-2,804 patients. Ann Surg. 2009;250(5):831-41.
18. Chang S, Laurent A, Tayar C, Karoui M, Cherqui D. Laparoscopy as a routine approach for left lateral sectionectomy. Br J Surg. 2007;94(1):58-63.
19. Kawaguchi Y, Fuks D, Kokudo N, Gayet B. Difficulty of laparoscopic liver resection. Ann Surg. 2018;267(1):13-7.
20. Ban D, Tanabe M, Ito H, Otsuka Y, Nitta H, Abe Y, et al. A novel difficulty scoring system for laparoscopic liver resection. J Hepatobiliary Pancreat Sci. 2014;21(10):745-53.
21. Halls MC, Berardi G, Cipriani F, Barkhatov L, Lainas P, Harris S, et al. Development and validation of a difficulty score to predict intraoperative complications during laparoscopic liver resection. Br J Surg. 2018;105(9):1182-91.
22. Wakabayashi G. What has changed after the Morioka consensus conference 2014 on laparoscopic liver resection? Hepatobiliary Surg Nutr. 2016;5(4):281-9.
23. Hasegawa Y, Wakabayashi G, Nitta H, Takahara T, Katagiri H, Umemura A, et al. A novel model for prediction of pure laparoscopic liver resection surgical difficulty. Surg Endosc. 2017;31(12):5356-63.
24. Ban D, Kudo A, Ito H, Mitsunori Y, Matsumura S, Aihara A, et al. The difficulty of laparoscopic liver resection. Updates Surg. 2015;67(2):123-8.
25. Tanaka S, Kawaguchi Y, Kubo S, Kanazawa A, Takeda Y, Hirokawa F, et al. Validation of index-based IWATE criteria as an improved difficulty scoring system for laparoscopic liver resection. Surg (United States). 2019;165(4):731-40.
26. Kawaguchi Y, Tanaka S, Fuks D, Kanazawa A, Takeda Y, Hirokawa F, et al. Validation and performance of three-level procedure-based classification for laparoscopic liver resection. Surg Endosc. 2020;34(5):2056-66.
27. Russolillo N, Maina C, Fleres F, Langella S, Lo Tesoriere R, Ferrero A. Comparison and validation of three difficulty scoring systems in laparoscopic liver surgery: a retrospective analysis on 300 cases. Surg Endosc. 2020;34(12):5484-94.
28. Hilal MA, Aldrighetti L, Dagher I, Edwin B, Troisi RI, Alikhanov R, et al. The Southampton Consensus Guidelines for laparoscopic liver surgery: from indication to implementation. Ann Surg. 2018;268(1):11-8.
29. Halls MC, Cipriani F, Berardi G, Barkhatov L, Lainas P, Alzoubi M, et al. Conversion for unfavorable intraoperative events results in significantly worst outcomes during laparoscopic liver resection: lessons learned from a multicenter review of 2861 cases. Ann Surg. 2018;268(6):1051-7.
30. Schiffman SC, Kim KH, Tsung A, Marsh JW, Geller DA. Laparoscopic versus open liver resection for metastatic colorectal cancer: a meta-analysis of 610 patients. Surg (United States). 2015;157(2):211-22.
31. Cheng Y, Zhang L, Li H, Wang L, Huang Y, Wu L, et al. Laparoscopic versus open liver resection for colorectal liver metastases: a systematic review. J Surg Res. 2017;220:234-46.

32. Zhang XL, Liu RF, Zhang D, Zhang YS, Wang T. Laparoscopic versus open liver resection for colorectal liver metastases: a systematic review and meta-analysis of studies with propensity score-based analysis. Int J Surg. 2017;44:191-203.
33. Hallet J, Beyfuss K, Memeo R, Karanicolas PJ, Marescaux J, Pessaux P. Short and long-term outcomes of laparoscopic compared to open liver resection for colorectal liver metastases. HepatoBiliary Surg Nutr. 2016;5(4):300-10.
34. Luo LX, Yu ZY, Bai YN. Laparoscopic hepatectomy for liver metastases from colorectal cancer: a meta-analysis. J Laparoendosc Adv Surg Tech. 2014;24(4):213-22.
35. Tian ZQ, Su XF, Lin ZY, Wu MC, Wei LX, He J. Meta-analysis of laparoscopic versus open liver resection for colorectal liver metastases. Oncotarget. 2016;7(51):84544-55.
36. Wei MT, He YZ, Wang JR, Chen N, Zhou ZG, Wang ZQ. Laparoscopic versus open hepatectomy with or without synchronous colectomy for colorectal liver metastasis: a meta-analysis. PLoS One. 2014;9(1):e87461.
37. Tranchart H, Fuks D, Vigano L, Ferretti S, Paye F, Wakabayashi G, et al. Laparoscopic simultaneous resection of colorectal primary tumor and liver metastases: a propensity score matching analysis. Surg Endosc. 2016;30(5):1853-62.
38. Castaing D, Vibert E, Ricca L, Azoulay D, Adam R, Gayet B. Oncologic results of laparoscopic versus open hepatectomy for colorectal liver metastases in two specialized centers. Ann Surg. 2009;250(5):849-55.
39. Fretland ÅA, Aghayan D, Edwin B. Long-term survival after laparoscopic versus open resection for colorectal liver metastases. J Clin Oncol. 2019;37(18_suppl):LBA3516.
40. Giulianotti PC, Coratti A, Angelini M, Sbrana F, Cecconi S, Balestracci T, et al. Robotics in general surgery: personal experience in a large community hospital. Arch Surg. 2003;138(7):777-84.
41. Kingham TP, Scherer MA, Neese BW, Clements LW, Stefansic JD, Jarnagin WR. Image guided liver surgery: intraoperative projection of computed tomography images utilizing tracked ultrasound. HPB. 2012;14(9):594-603.
42. Casciola L, Patriti A, Ceccarelli G, Bartoli A, Ceribelli C, Spaziani A. Robot-assisted parenchymal-sparing liver surgery including lesions located in the posterosuperior segments. Surg Endosc. 2011;25(12):3815-24.
43. Di Benedetto F, Tarantino G, Magistri P. Chasing the right path: tips, tricks and challenges of robotic approach to posterior segments. Hepatobiliary Surg Nutr. 2019;8(5):512-4.
44. Montalti R, Scuderi V, Patriti A, Vivarelli M, Troisi RI. Robotic versus laparoscopic resections of posterosuperior segments of the liver: a propensity score-matched comparison. Surg Endosc. 2016;30(3):1004-13.
45. Qiu J, Chen S, Chengyou D. A systematic review of robotic-assisted liver resection and meta-analysis of robotic versus laparoscopic hepatectomy for hepatic neoplasms. Surg Endosc. 2016;30(3):862-75.
46. Troisi RI, Patriti A, Montalti R, Casciola L. Robot assistance in liver surgery: a real advantage over a fully laparoscopic approach? Results of a comparative bi-institutional analysis. Int J Med Robot Comput Assist Surg. 2013;9(2):160-6.
47. Beppu T, Wakabayashi G, Hasegawa K, Gotohda N, Mizuguchi T, Takahashi Y, et al. Long-term and perioperative outcomes of laparoscopic versus open liver resection for colorectal liver metastases with propensity score matching: a multi-institutional Japanese study. J Hepatobiliary Pancreat Sci. 2015;22(10):711-20.

48. Fretland AA, Dagenborg VJ, Bjørnelv GMW, Kazaryan AM, Kristiansen R, Fagerland MW, et al. Laparoscopic versus open resection for colorectal liver metastases. Ann Surg. 2018;267(2):199-207.
49. Fuks D, Nomi T, Ogiso S, Gelli M, Velayutham V, Conrad C, et al. Laparoscopic two-stage hepatectomy for bilobar colorectal liver metastases. Br J Surg. 2015;102(13):1684-90.
50. Aghayan DL, Pelanis E, Avdem Fretland Å, Kazaryan AM, Sahakyan MA, Røsok BI, et al. Laparoscopic parenchyma-sparing liver resection for colorectal metastases. Radiol Oncol. 2018;52(1):36-41.
51. Dagher I, O'Rourke N, Geller DA, Cherqui D, Belli G, Gamblin TC, et al. Laparoscopic major hepatectomy: an evolution in standard of care. Ann Surg. 2009;250(5):856-60.
52. Nomi T, Fuks D, Kawaguchi Y, Mal F, Nakajima Y, Gayet B. Learning curve for laparoscopic major hepatectomy. Br J Surg. 2015;102(7):796-804.
53. Gayet B, Cavaliere D, Vibert E, Perniceni T, Levard H, Denet C, et al. Totally laparoscopic right hepatectomy. Am J Surg. 2007;194(5):685-9.
54. Hilal MA, Fabio F Di, Teng MJ, Lykoudis P, Primrose JN, Pearce NW. Single-centre comparative study of laparoscopic versus open right hepatectomy. J Gastrointest Surg. 2011;15(5):818-23.
55. Takahara T, Wakabayashi G, Konno H, Gotoh M, Yamaue H, Yanaga K, et al. Comparison of laparoscopic major hepatectomy with propensity score matched open cases from the National Clinical Database in Japan. J Hepatobiliary Pancreat Sci. 2016;23(11):721-34.
56. Pattaro G, Fuks D, Tranchart H, Ettorre GM, Suhool A, Bourdeaux C, et al. Laparoscopic left liver resections: how far can we go? Surg Endosc Other Interv Tech. 2017;31(12):5303-11.
57. Kasai M, Cipriani F, Gayet B, Aldrighetti L, Ratti F, Sarmiento JM, et al. Laparoscopic versus open major hepatectomy: a systematic review and meta-analysis of individual patient data. Surg (United States). 2018;163(5):985-95.
58. De Blasi V, Memeo R, Adam R, Goéré D, Cherqui D, Regimbeau JM, et al. Major hepatectomy for colorectal liver metastases in patients aged over 80: a propensity score matching analysis. Dig Surg. 2018;35(4):333-41.
59. Gumbs AA, Bar-Zakai B, Gayet B. Totally laparoscopic extended left hepatectomy. J Gastrointest Surg. 2008;12(7):1152.
60. Gumbs AA, Gayet B. Multimedia article. Totally laparoscopic extended right hepatectomy. Surg Endosc. 2008;22(9):2076-7.
61. Pietrasz D, Fuks D, Subar D, Donatelli G, Ferretti C, Lamer C, et al. Laparoscopic extended liver resection: are postoperative outcomes different? Surg Endosc. 2018;32(12):4833-40.
62. Halls MC, Alseidi A, Berardi G, Cipriani F, Van der Poel M, Davila D, et al. A comparison of the learning curves of laparoscopic liver surgeons in differing stages of the IDEAL paradigm of surgical innovation: standing on the shoulders of pioneers. Ann Surg. 2019;269(2):221-8.
63. Coles SR, Besselink MG, Serin KR, Alsaati H, Di Gioia P, Samim M, et al. Total laparoscopic management of lesions involving liver segment 7. Surg Endosc. 2015;29(11):3190-5.
64. Martínez-Cecilia D, Fontana M, Siddiqi NN, Halls M, Barbaro S, Abu-Hilal M. Laparoscopic parenchymal sparing resections in segment 8: techniques for a demanding and infrequent procedure. Surg Endosc. 2018;29(11):3190-5.

65. Scuderi V, Barkhatov L, Montalti R, Ratti F, Cipriani F, Pardo F, et al. Outcome after laparoscopic and open resections of posterosuperior segments of the liver. Br J Surg. 2017; 104(6):751-9.
66. Garbarino GM, Marchese U, Tobome R, Ward MA, Vibert E, Gayet B, et al. Laparoscopic versus open unisegmentectomy in two specialized centers. Feasibility and short-term results. HPB. 2019;2020;22(5):750-6.
67. Zheng H, Huang SG, Qin SM, Xiang F. Comparison of laparoscopic versus open liver resection for lesions located in posterosuperior segments: a meta-analysis of short-term and oncological outcomes. Surg Endosc. 2019;33(12):3910-8.
68. Del Pino S, Fischer L, Nashan B, Li J. Reduced opioid-demand and fewer pulmonary complications after laparoscopic liver resection in the posterior segments. Dig Surg. 2020;37(2):129-34.
69. Cipriani F, Ratti F, Paganelli M, Reineke R, Catena M, Aldrighetti L. Laparoscopic or open approaches for posterosuperior and anterolateral liver resections? A propensity score based analysis of the degree of advantage. HPB. 2019;21(12):1676-86.
70. De Jong MC, Pulitano C, Ribero D, Strub J, Mentha G, Schulick RD, et al. Rates and patterns of recurrence following curative intent surgery for colorectal liver metastasis: an international multi- institutional analysis of 1669 patients. Ann Surg. 2009;250(3):440-8.
71. Wicherts DA, De Haas RJ, Salloum C, Andreani P, Pascal G, Sotirov D, et al. Repeat hepatectomy for recurrent colorectal metastases. Br J Surg. 2013;100(6):808-18.
72. Adam R, Pascal G, Azoulay D, Tanaka K, Castaing D, Bismuth H, et al. Liver resection for colorectal metastases: the third hepatectomy. Ann Surg. 2003; 238(6):871-83.
73. Shaw IM, Rees M, Welsh FKS, Bygrave S, John TG. Repeat hepatic resection for recurrent colorectal liver metastases is associated with favourable long-term survival. Br J Surg. 2006;93(4):457-64.
74. Ou Ounhu A, Laurent O, Rault A, Coudere D, Nullier E, Carie J. A second liver resection due to recurrent colorectal liver metastases. Arch Surg. 2007;142(12): 1144-9.
75. Adam R, Wicherts DA, De Haas R, Ciacio O, Levi F, Paule B, et al. Patients with initially unresectable colorectal liver metastases: is there a possibility of cure? J Clin Oncol. 2009;27(11):1829-35.
76. De Haas RJ, Wicherts DA, Flores E, Azoulay D, Castaing D, Adam R. R1 resection by necessity for colorectal liver metastases: is it still a contraindication to surgery? Ann Surg. 2008;248(4):626-37.
77. Yamazaki S, Takayama T, Okada S, Iwama A, Midorikawa Y, Moriguchi M, et al. Good candidates for a third liver resection of colorectal metastasis. World J Surg. 2013;37(4):847-53.
78. Nomi T, Fuks D, Ogiso S, Nakajima Y, Louvet C, Gayet B. Second and third laparoscopic liver resection for patients with recurrent colorectal liver metastases. Ann Surg. 2016;263(5):e68-72.
79. van der Poel MJ, Barkhatov L, Fuks D, Berardi G, Cipriani F, Aljaiuossi A, et al. Multicentre propensity score-matched study of laparoscopic versus open repeat liver resection for colorectal liver metastases. Br J Surg. 2019;106(6):783-9.
80. Kamarajah SK, Bundred J, Manas D, Jiao LR, Hilal MA, White SA. Robotic versus conventional laparoscopic liver resections: a systematic review and meta-analysis. Scand J Surg. 2021;110(3):290-300.

CHAPTER

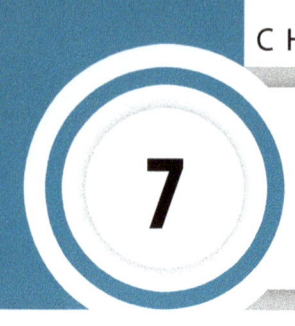

Minimally Invasive Surgery in Gallbladder Carcinoma

Yugal Limbu, Sujan Regmee, Roshan Ghimire

▮ INTRODUCTION

The use of minimally invasive surgery (MIS) in managing gastrointestinal tract cancers has come a long way since its beginning. Due to concerns regarding tumor cell dissemination and fears of incomplete tumor removal, MIS for gastric and colonic cancers, which is now standard of care, was looked upon with reservation in the past.[1,2] However, the use of laparoscopic and robotic surgery for managing gallbladder cancer (GBC) is still a matter of debate among experts across the globe. The port site recurrence and bile spillage that may cause tumor dissemination have been concerns of hepatobiliary surgeons. Moreover, the technical difficulty of laparoscopic liver resection (LLR) and lymph node (LN) dissection around the hepatoduodenal ligament have hindered adopting the minimally invasive approach for GBC.[3] Although MIS for extended cholecystectomies for GBC has been contraindicated in the past, recent studies have demonstrated that laparoscopic surgery does not adversely affect the perioperative and survival outcomes of patients with GBC.[4-8]

▮ PREOPERATIVE WORKUP

Before surgery, a thorough preoperative workup to determine the depth of invasion is pivotal to determining the best surgical approach and patient prognosis. Compared to transabdominal ultrasound and contrast-enhanced computed tomography, endoscopic and laparoscopic ultrasound have higher resolution and thus are more precise to determine the T staging of the tumor.[9,10] Using multimodality imaging for precise staging improves clinical and survival outcomes in patients undergoing surgery for GBC.[4,11]

▮ LAPAROSCOPIC SURGERY FOR SUSPECTED T1a TUMORS

In the past, open surgery was recommended even for suspected early-stage GBC because of the abovementioned concerns regarding MIS. However, studies have shown that MIS does not adversely influence the prognosis of patients with early-stage GBC. Furthermore, when definitive oncologic resection is performed for GBC detected incidentally during surgery or diagnosed postoperatively, survival is not adversely affected by laparoscopic surgery.[12,13] Nevertheless, some studies show adverse survival outcomes in incidentally diagnosed GBC following laparoscopic surgery for acute cholecystitis. Therefore, laparoscopic surgery may be better indicated for GBC that is not associated with acute cholecystitis.

LAPAROSCOPIC EXTENDED CHOLECYSTECTOMY FOR T1b AND ABOVE TUMORS

The extent of surgery in patients with GBC varies based on clinical presentation and the nature of the tumor that can range from a small polypoid mass to a sizeable mass invading the GB bed, hilum of the liver, or other adjacent organs. In recent reports, the indications for laparoscopic extended cholecystectomy (defined as cholecystectomy + dissection of regional LNs ± liver resection inclusive of the GB bed) have been primarily for stage T1 and T2 GBC. However, evidence to support this procedure for stage T3 GBC is limited.

The goals of radical surgery for GBC are adequate LN dissection, margin-free liver resection, and bile duct resection/reconstruction when needed. These goals have been safely achieved using minimally invasive techniques in various studies.[3-6,8,14-18] Liver resection is recommended in tumors T1b and above tumors to achieve a negative resection margin on the hepatic side and minimize the likelihood of recurrence by removing microscopic metastases in the liver. MIS procedures for GBC include wedge liver resection or segment IVb/V bi-segmentectomy with LN dissection, and these two techniques are comparable in terms of safety and survival outcome.[19] Laparoscopic bile duct resection can be performed when cystic duct margin is positive or when the tumor involves the bile duct.[15-18]

Although the extent of LN dissection during radical surgery for GBC is debated, there is consensus among experts to remove the LNs around the hepatoduodenal ligament **(Fig. 1)**. Moreover, LNs in the posterior-superior pancreaticoduodenal area and along the common hepatic artery are also removed routinely in some centers, including ours, due to frequent metastasis to these regions.[20,21]

According to American Joint Committee on Cancer (AJCC), 8th edition TNM classification, at least six LNs are necessary for adequate lymphatic clearance, which is safely achieved using a laparoscopic approach.[7,12,13,22] Aortocaval LN sampling for a frozen section at the initiation of surgery is recommended in selected cases because its involvement renders the tumor unresectable and the patient not subjected to radical surgery.[8]

INDICATION FOR BILE DUCT RESECTION IN LAPAROSCOPIC EXTENDED CHOLECYSTECTOMY

Bile duct resection is not routinely performed for LN clearance because of increased morbidity associated with the procedure without any significant

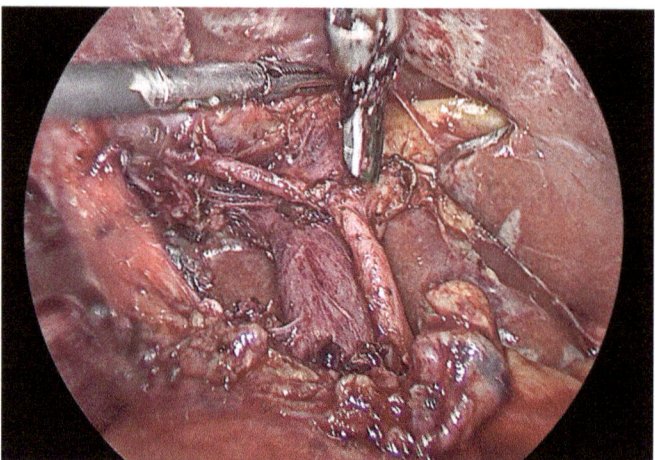

Fig. 1: Lymphatic clearance of hepatoduodenal ligament.

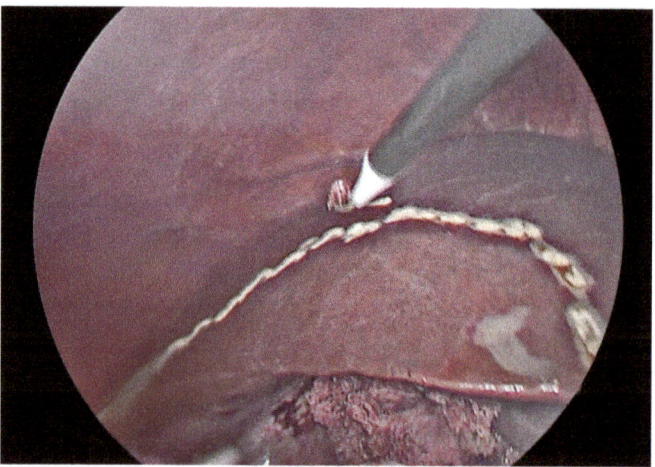

Fig. 2: Laparoscopic marking for non-anatomical segmental resection.

survival benefit.[19,20] However, bile duct resection is warranted when the cystic duct margin is positive, or there is direct tumor invasion of the bile duct. Studies have shown that laparoscopic bile duct excision for GBC can be safely performed with clinical outcomes comparable to open surgery.[14,16-18]

Although the evidence is limited, the recurrence and survival rates were found to be similar between laparoscopic and open surgery groups in comparative studies.[6,14]

LAPAROSCOPIC EXTENDED CHOLECYSTECTOMY IN THE INCIDENTALLY DIAGNOSED GALLBLADDER

Incidental GBC is reported in 0.19–3.3% of cases following laparoscopic cholecystectomy for symptomatic gallstone disease.[23] Due to postoperative

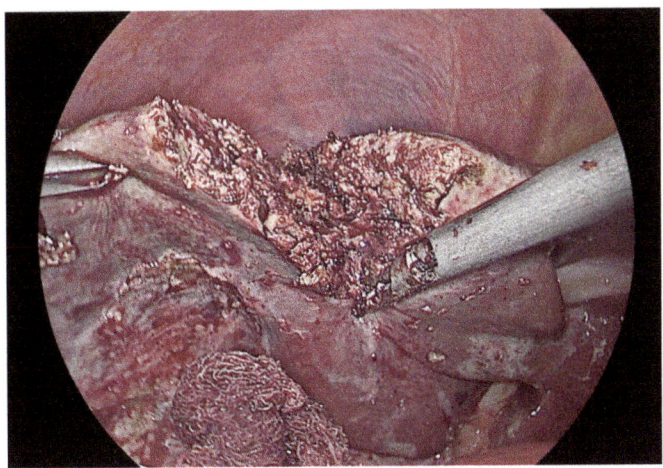

Fig. 3: Liver resection with use of Harmonic Scalpel Ò.

inflammatory adhesions and fibrosis around the hepatoduodenal ligament, the second operation is usually conducted using an open technique. However, many studies support the use of the laparoscopic technique for definitive surgery following incidental CGB.[6,8,15,17,22] Moreover, unlike first surgery for GBC, laparoscopic reoperation is not associated with the risk of tumor seeding related to bile spillage as there is no gallbladder **(Figs. 2 and 3)**. Therefore, a laparoscopic approach for incidental is acceptable, with a comparable clinical and oncological outcome.

Previously, in postoperatively diagnosed GBC, port-site metastasis was a concern, however, studies show that port site metastasis indicates disseminated disease rather than iatrogenic tumor dissemination. Routine port-site resection is not associated with improved survival or reduced recurrence and therefore is not routinely recommended during the definitive surgical treatment.[24]

■ ROBOTIC SURGERY IN GALLBLADDER CANCER

The robotic approach has been used in extended cholecystectomy for the past few years. Its primary steps are divided into two parts: gallbladder resection along with the segment of liver and regional LN dissection. The patient is kept in 45° reverse Trendelenburg position for this procedure to allow the small bowel and the transverse colon to be displaced away from the operating site. A straight line is drawn from the anterior superior iliac spine to a point below the umbilicus, and three 8-mm robotic ports are placed. The fourth robotic port is placed slightly above the remaining three ports in the imaginary line between the umbilicus and the left subcostal margin. A 12-mm assistant port is placed. The camera is placed through the second or third port, and the other ports are used as working ports. Standard surgical procedure is performed, similar to laparoscopic surgery sticking to the basic principles of surgery of gallbladder carcinoma. The robotic procedure provides a precise three-dimensional image of the operative field, improves dexterity, and eliminates hand vibration, making the surgery more precise.[25,26] This provides a clear advantage above the laparoscopic procedure. The first robotic extended cholecystectomy was reported by Shen et al.[27] in 2002; five patients were included in his series, showing that the procedure is safe and feasible.

Published reports have shown that robotic extended cholecystectomy patients had less intraoperative blood loss and shorter postoperative hospital stay.[28,29] For a good oncological surgery, LN yield is essential. The LN yield was reported to be >10 in number in the series published by Goel et al. The conversion rate reported for major hepatobiliary robotic surgery is 3.7–47%,[30] and a learning curve of 10–13 cases were reported in a study published by Tsung et al.[31]

In conclusion, the use of laparoscopic and robotic approaches to manage selected cases of GBC is safe and feasible in specialized centers with adequate experience in hepatobiliary and MIS.

REFERENCES

1. Lacy AM, García-Valdecasas JC, Delgado S, Castells A, Taurá P, M Piqué J, et al. Laparoscopy-assisted colectomy versus open colectomy for treatment of non-metastatic colon cancer: a randomised trial. Lancet. 2002;359(9325):2224-9.
2. Yüksel C, Erşen O, Mercan Ü, Başçeken SI, Bakırarar B, Bayar S, et al. Long-term results and current problems in laparoscopic gastrectomy: single-center experience. J Laparoendosc Adv Surg Tech. 2020;30(11):1204-14.
3. D'Silva M, Han HS, Yoon YS, Cho JY. Minimally invasive liver resection for gallbladder cancer. Laparosc Surg. 2021;5(4).
4. Cho JY, Han HS, Yoon YS, Ahn KS, Kim YH, Lee KH. Laparoscopic approach for suspected early-stage gallbladder carcinoma. Arch Surg. 2010;145(2):128-33.
5. Lee SE, Jang JY, Lim CS, Kang MJ, Kim SW. Systematic review on the surgical treatment for T1 gallbladder cancer. World J Gastroenterol. 2011;17(2):174-80.
6. Agarwal AK, Javed A, Kalayarasan R, Sakhuja P. Minimally invasive versus the conventional open surgical approach of a radical cholecystectomy for gallbladder cancer: a retrospective comparative study. HPB. 2015;17(6):536-41.
7. Gumbs AA, Jarufe N, Gayet B. Minimally invasive approaches to extrapancreatic cholangiocarcinoma. Surg. Endosc. 2013;27(2):406-14.
8. Shirobe T, Maruyama S. Laparoscopic radical cholecystectomy with lymph node dissection for gallbladder carcinoma. Surg Endosc. 2015;29(8):2244-50.
9. Jang JY, Kim SW, Lee SE, Wook Hwang DW, Kim EJ, Lee JY, et al. Differential diagnostic and staging accuracies of high resolution ultrasonography, endoscopic ultrasonography, and multidetector computed tomography for gallbladder polypoid lesions and gallbladder cancer. Ann Surg. 2009;250(6):943-9.
10. Fujita N, Noda Y, Kobayashi G, Kimura K, Yago A. Diagnosis of the depth of invasion of gallbladder carcinoma by EUS. Gastrointest Endosc. 1999;50(5):659-63.

11. Yoon YS, Han HS, Cho JY, Choi Y, Lee W, Jang JY, et al. Is laparoscopy contraindicated for gallbladder cancer? A 10-year prospective cohort study. J Am Coll Surg. 2015;221(4):847-53.
12. Whalen GF, Bird I, Tanski W, Russell JC, Clive J. Laparoscopic cholecystectomy does not demonstrably decrease survival of patients with serendipitously treated gallbladder cancer. J Am Coll Surg. 2001;192(2):189-95.
13. Ouchi K, Mikuni J, Kakugawa Y. Laparoscopic cholecystectomy for gallbladder carcinoma: Results of a Japanese survey of 498 patients. J Hepatobiliary Pancreat Surg. 2002;9(2):256-60.
14. Itano O, Oshima G, Minagawa T, Shinoda M, Kitago M, Abe Y, et al. Novel strategy for laparoscopic treatment of pT2 gallbladder carcinoma. Surg Endosc. 2015;29(12):3600-7.
15. Palanisamy S, Patel N, Sabnis S, Palanisamy N, Vijay A, Palanivelu P, et al. Laparoscopic radical cholecystectomy for suspected early gall bladder carcinoma: thinking beyond convention. Surg Endosc. 2016;30(6):2442-8.
16. Gumbs AA, Hoffman JP. Laparoscopic radical cholecystectomy and Roux-en-Y choledochojejunostomy for gallbladder cancer. Surg Endosc. 2010;24(7):1766-8.
17. Gumbs AA, Milone L, Geha R, Delacroix J, Chabot JA. Laparoscopic radical cholecystectomy. J Laparoendosc Adv Surg Tech. 2009;19(4):519-20.
18. Machado MA, Makdissi FF, Surjan RC. Totally laparoscopic hepatic bisegmentectomy (s4b+s5) and hilar lymphadenectomy for incidental gallbladder cancer. Ann Surg Oncol. 2015;22:336-9.
19. Yu LH, Yuan B, Fu XH, Yu WL, Liu J, Zhang YJ. Does anatomic resection get more benefits than wedge hepatectomy on the prognosis for pT3 unsuspected gallbladder cancer? J Laparoendosc Adv Surg Tech. 2019;29(11):1414-8.
20. Miyazaki M, Yoshitomi H, Miyakawa S, Uesaka K, Unno M, Endo I, et al. Clinical practice guidelines for the management of biliary tract cancers 2015: the 2nd English edition. J Hepatobiliary Pancreat Sci. 2015;22(4):249-73.
21. Chijiiwa K, Noshiro H, Nakano K, Okido M, Sugitani A, Yamaguchi K, et al. Role of surgery for gallbladder carcinoma with special reference to lymph node metastasis and stage using western and Japanese classification systems. World J Surg. 2000;24(10):1271-7.
22. Maharjan DK, Thapa PB. Laparoscopic extended cholecystectomy for early gall bladder cancer. J Nepal Health Res Counc. 2021;18(4):724-8.
23. Sujata J, Rana S, Sabina K, Hassan MJ, Zeeba SJ. Incidental gall bladder carcinoma in laparoscopic cholecystectomy: a report of 6 cases and a review of the literature. J Clin Diagnostic Res. 2013;7(1):85-8.
24. Ethun CG, Postlewait LM, Le N, Pawlik TM, Poultsides G, Tran T, et al. Routine port-site excision in incidentally discovered gallbladder cancer is not associated with improved survival: a multi-institution analysis from the US Extrahepatic Biliary Malignancy Consortium. J Surg Oncol. 2017;115(7):805-11.
25. Lai ECH, Yang GPC, Tang CN. Robot-assisted laparoscopic liver resection for hepatocellular carcinoma: short-term outcome. Am J Surg. 2013;205(6):697-702.
26. Szold A, Bergamaschi R, Broeders I, Dankelman J, Forgione A, Langø T, et al. European Association of Endoscopic Surgeons (EAES) consensus statement on the use of robotics in general surgery. Surg Endosc. 2015;29(2):253-88.
27. Shen BY, Zhan Q, Deng XX, Bo H, Liu Q, Peng CH, et al. Radical resection of gallbladder cancer: could it be robotic? Surg Endosc. 2012;26(11):3245-50.

28. Georgakis GV, Novak S, Bartlett DL, Zureikat AH, Zeh HJ, Hogg ME. The emerging role of minimally-invasive surgery for gallbladder cancer: a comparison to open surgery. Conn Med. 2018;82(4):211-6.
29. Goel M, Khobragade K, Patkar S, Kanetkar A, Kurunkar S. Robotic surgery for gallbladder cancer: operative technique and early outcomes. J Surg Oncol. 2019;119(7):958-63.
30. Giulianotti PC, Bianco FM, Daskalaki D, Gonzalez-Ciccarelli LF, Kim J, Benedetti E. Robotic liver surgery: technical aspects and review of the literature. Hepatobiliary Surg Nutr. 2016;5(4):311-21.
31. Tsung A, Geller DA, Sukato DC, Sabbaghian S, Tohme S, Steel J, et al. Robotic versus laparoscopic hepatectomy: a matched comparison. Ann Surg. 2014;259(3):549-55.

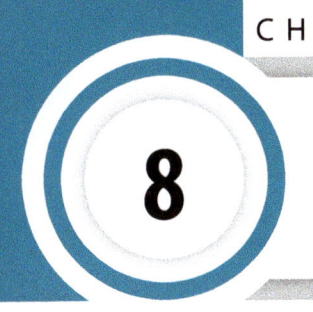

CHAPTER 8

Changing Trends in Minimal Invasive Pancreatic Surgery

Savio George Barreto

■ INTRODUCTION

Minimally invasive surgery has transformed general surgical practice tremendously over the last three decades. However, the adoption of laparoscopic surgery has been slower than other fields of general surgery. The reasons for this are obvious once the complexity of pancreatic surgery is considered, namely, the anatomical location (in the retroperitoneum) and (major vascular) relations of the gland, the need to reconstruct (as in the case of pancreatoduodenectomy/PD), limited degree of freedom of movement with conventional laparoscopic instruments, two-dimensional vision, and the inherent morbidity associated with pancreatic surgery in the perioperative period.[1] However, despite these hurdles, pancreatic surgeons, appreciating the benefits of minimally invasive surgery, continue to soldier on looking for opportunities to adopt this approach with a view to advancing the field, yet not losing focus that it is the interests of the patient that trump any approach even if it is considered an advancement in technology.

This chapter will present the reader with an overview of the evolution of minimally invasive pancreatic surgery from its humble beginnings as a diagnostic procedure more than a century ago to laparoscopic and robotic PD. In doing so, the arguments for, and against, minimally invasive pancreatic surgery will be presented. This will leave the reader with an understanding of where the evidence in literature, as well as the fraternity currently stand in terms of minimally invasive pancreatic surgery.

■ IT ALL BEGAN WITH ORGANOSCOPY....

Bernheim published his experience with diagnostic laparoscopy for pancreatic diseases using a cystoscope in 1911.[2] This was followed by a hiatus in published literature through the two world wars with the next reports for the same procedure only surfacing in the 1970s.[3,4]

The credit for pioneering resectional minimally invasive pancreatic surgery goes to Gagner and Pomp who reported in 1994[5] the first laparoscopic pylorus-preserving PD performed for a patient with chronic pancreatitis (CP) who incidentally had pancreas divisum. They followed this report by a series of six patients[6] on whom they successfully performed laparoscopic distal pancreatectomies (DPs) and enucleations on for islet cell tumors with reasonable postoperative outcomes. Thereafter, there was a steady increase in the number of minimally invasive surgeries especially for DPs and enucleations for benign tumors given the improved vision and lack of need for reconstruction/anastomoses. The acceptance of minimally invasive pancreatic surgery for malignant lesions was not as overwhelming owing to the concerns of implantation of malignant cells into laparoscopic port-sites because of aerosolization and dissemination due to the pneumoperitoneum and also from the trocars leading to port-site metastases[7,8] as well as the issue of radicality of the operation.

In 2003, Giulianotti et al.[9] reported the first experience with robotic pancreatic surgery. The authors reported performing eight PDs and five DPs. Of the eight patients who underwent PDs, in six of them, the surgeons performed a hybrid procedure comprising a laparoscopic resection and robotics used for the bilioenteric anastomosis and gastroenterostomy. It appeared that in none of the patients was a pancreaticoenteric anastomosis fashioned with the duct opening on the remnant sealed off with glue. The mortality rate was 12.5%.

Minimally invasive surgery even has a role in the infected pancreatic necrosis. Acknowledging the surgical stress to the patient with repeated open necrosectomies, Carter, McKay, and Imrie not only described percutaneous necrosectomy[10] but pioneered the now established doctrine of the "step-up" approach for infected pancreatic necrosis made famous by the PANTER trial.[11]

Over the last decade, there have been numerous large series and even randomized controlled trials comparing open versus minimally invasive surgery and even comparing laparoscopic to robotic surgery. I will address the concept of changing trends in minimally invasive pancreatic surgery using a series of questions, namely:

- Is minimally invasive pancreatic surgery feasible and safe?
- Is minimally invasive pancreatic surgery an oncologically viable option for adenocarcinoma of the pancreas?
- What are the evidence-based indications for minimally invasive pancreatic surgery today?
- Is robotics more advantageous to laparoscopic DP?
- Is minimally invasive surgery cost-effective?
- How easy is it to train in minimally invasive pancreatic surgery?
- Are we doing our patients a disservice if we do not offer them minimally invasive pancreatic surgery?

Is Minimally Invasive Pancreatic Surgery Feasible and Safe?

Minimally invasive diagnostic laparoscopy, DP, and necrosectomy are feasible and safe when performed by trained surgeons and for the right indications.[12] While minimally invasive PD is feasible, its safety remains a matter of concern even in the hands of expert, trained surgeons.[13] It must be stressed here that the published data on minimally invasive surgery is from high-volume centers and from high-volume surgeons and this needs to be factored in when interpreting the evidence in literature and determining its implementation in a surgeon's own practice.

Is Minimally Invasive Pancreatic Surgery an Oncologically Viable Option for Adenocarcinoma of the Pancreas?

The most updated and unbiased analysis of the literature on the oncological safety/equivalence of minimally invasive versus open DP failed to satisfactorily answer this question in the absence of data with long-term follow-up from randomized controlled trials.[14] The author's impression of the perceived advantage of laparoscopic DP over open in terms of a reduced hospital stay was that these data are derived from observational studies from centers performing laparoscopic surgeries on patients not necessarily comparable to those undergoing open surgery. Thus, in the case of pancreatic cancer, we are unable to confidently confirm, nor dispute the oncological safety of minimally invasive surgery at the present time. However, this question will likely be answered once the long-term results of the randomized controlled trials[13,15,16] comparing open versus minimally invasive DP and PD for cancer become available.

What are the Evidence-based Indications for Minimally Invasive Pancreatic Surgery Today?

The current indications in which minimally invasive pancreatic surgery has been found to be comparable, or maybe even advantageous, to open surgery include the following:

Acute Necrotizing Pancreatitis

Minimally invasive retroperitoneal necrosectomy is a preferred option in patients with infected pancreatic necrosis extending to the left flank and in whom percutaneous drainage has failed to control sepsis, a necrosectomy is warranted, and clear access to the pancreatic bed is available. This approach is indicated when open surgery is either not required to drain multiple other collections, deal with a perforated or obstructed bowel, reduce intra-abdominal pressure, or secure a feeding access.

Benign Pancreatic Tumors

Minimally invasive DP is preferred, whenever feasible, for benign and low-grade malignant tumors over open DP given its proven advantages that include a reduced hospital stay, intraoperative blood loss, and complication rates that are not different from open surgery.[12]

Staging of Pancreatic Cancer

The main indication for staging laparoscopy with or without ultrasonography is in the assessment of patients with nonmetastatic, locally advanced or borderline resectable tumors based on conventional radiology.[17] Other indications include patients with a high serum carbohydrate antigen/CA 19-9 level, cancers with large regional lymph nodes, and in cancers of the body and tail.[18] When performed for these indications, staging laparoscopy can either detect occult liver and/or peritoneal metastases with sensitivities approaching 88 and 93%, respectively,[19] or confirm the nonmetastatic nature of the cancer helping to appropriately direct the patients toward neoadjuvant therapy.[20] If staging laparoscopy and ultrasonography is used in all patients with pancreatic cancer, it is correctly able to predict resectability in 79% compared to 55% on conventional imaging. It is thus useful in avoiding noncurative laparotomies, with their attendant morbidity, in 33% of patients.[21]

Is Robotics More Advantageous than Laparoscopic Distal Pancreatectomy?

Robotic DP is feasible and as safe as laparoscopic DP.[22] It offers no additional advantage in comparison to laparoscopic DP. Thus, the choice between robotic versus laparoscopic DP for benign and low-grade malignant tumors should be based on the surgeons' experience and local resources available.[12]

Is Minimally Invasive Surgery Cost-effective?

It was previously believed that minimally invasive pancreatic surgery is expensive (owing to the expensive consumables and significantly longer operating time) and this was considered a drawback of the technique. However, a combined analysis of all studies relating to perioperative costs have shown that while it is true that the operative costs are higher for minimally invasive pancreatic surgery, these increased expenses are offset by the fact that postoperative recovery is enhanced and the proportion of complications is comparable to open surgery.[23] Enhanced recovery (clinical care pathways) programs following pancreatectomy have not only been shown to reduce hospital stay,[24] but also costs.[25] It is worth noting here that there are no studies comparing costs following minimally invasive versus open surgery (with enhanced recovery protocols in place). Additionally, given that the equivalence of costs between laparoscopic, robotic, and open surgery may not be uniform all over the world,[26,27] it would be prudent for national audits to be conducted to determine the actual economic situation within a particular healthcare system instead of extrapolating data from other systems.

How Easy is it to Train in Minimally Invasive Pancreatic Surgery?

It is evident from all the above that minimally invasive surgery has a role in the surgical management of pancreatic diseases and this role is being clarified with accumulating evidence. Thus, being trained in minimally invasive pancreatic surgery is an important skill set for pancreatic surgeons, especially those working in countries where minimally invasive is accessible. Similar to open pancreatic surgery, minimally invasive pancreatic surgery has a significant learning curve and participation in dedicated training programs with sufficient volume is warranted for its safe implementation.[28] For laparoscopic distal pancreatectomy, the learning curve is 30 cases,[29] while 40 cases are required for the achievement of technical competence in laparoscopic PD and 100 cases to obtain the skill set to address highly challenging cases.[30] In the case of robotic DP, the learning curve is between 20 and 40 cases to develop competence when assessing operating time and readmission rate.[31] It is important to provide context when interpreting these data. These learning curves have been generated at high-volume centers by surgeons competent in open pancreatic surgery. Thus, surgeons willing to train in minimally invasive pancreatic resectional surgery must be competent in open pancreatic surgery and must look to be trained at accredited high-volume centers.[28]

ARE WE DOING OUR PATIENTS A DISSERVICE IF WE DO NOT OFFER THEM MINIMALLY INVASIVE PANCREATIC SURGERY?

What can be gleaned from the available evidence in literature largely originating from high-volume centers of excellence for pancreatic surgery is that minimally invasive pancreatic surgery is feasible and safe when performed for the correct indications. It has certainly been a valued addition to the armamentarium of the pancreatic surgeon.[32] It has its advantages, the most important being enhanced recovery. It must be pointed out, though, that the evidence favoring minimally invasive surgery does not extend to PD.[33] Interestingly, the adoption of clinical care pathways[24] targeting enhanced-recovery after pancreatic surgery has been shown to be successful even for open PD.[34] Universal adoption of these protocols must be encouraged irrespective of whether the patient undergoes open or minimally invasive surgery. Pancreatic surgery, open or minimally invasive, is fraught with a high risk of morbidity and even the possible risk of mortality.[35,36] To this day, pancreatic surgeons continue to battle the significant complications of resectional surgery[37-39] as well as life-threatening, infected pancreatic necrosis following severe AP.[40] Minimally invasive surgery, in the best of hands, provides outcomes comparable to open surgery. Surgeons must consider training in minimally invasive pancreatic surgery to expand their skill set and provide their patients the option of minimally invasive surgery, when indicated. However, delivering quality care by trained pancreatic surgeons is the need of the hour irrespective of whether this therapy is being administered by the open, or minimally invasive (laparoscopic or robotic), approach.

REFERENCES

1. Shrikhande SV, Barreto SG, Shukla PJ. Laparoscopy in pancreatic tumors. J Minim Access Surg. 2007;3(2):47-51.
2. Bernheim BM. IV. Organoscopy: cystoscopy of the abdominal cavity. Ann Surg. 1911;53(6):764-7.
3. Cuschieri A, Hall AW, Clark J. Value of laparoscopy in the diagnosis and management of pancreatic carcinoma. Gut. 1978;19(7):672-7.
4. Meyer-Burg J, Ziegler U, Palme G. Supragastric pancreascopy. Results of 125 laparoscopies. Dtsch Med Wochenschr. 1972;97:1969-72.
5. Gagner M, Pomp A. Laparoscopic pylorus-preserving pancreatoduodenectomy. Surg Endosc. 1994;8(5):408-10.
6. Gagner M, Pomp A, Herrera MF. Early experience with laparoscopic resections of islet cell tumors. Surgery. 1996;120(6):1051-4.
7. Hopkins MP, Dulai RM, Occhino A, Holda S. The effects of carbon dioxide pneumoperitoneum on seeding of tumor in port sites in a rat model. Am J Obstet Gynecol. 1999;181(6):1329-33; discussion 33-4.
8. Shukla PJ, Barreto SG, Shrikhande SV, Mohandas M, Nilendu P, Venkatesh R, et al. Detection of gall bladder cancer metastases in rare sites by PET scan. Indian J Gastroenterol. 2007;26(6):303-4.
9. Giulianotti PC, Coratti A, Angelini M, Sbrana F, Cecconi S, Balestracci T, et al. Robotics in general surgery: personal experience in a large community hospital. Arch Surg. 2003;138(7):777-84.
10. Carter CR, McKay CJ, Imrie CW. Percutaneous necrosectomy and sinus tract endoscopy in the management of infected pancreatic necrosis: an initial experience. Ann Surg. 2000;232(2):175-80.
11. van Santvoort HC, Besselink MG, Bakker OJ, Hofker HS, Boermeester MA, Dejong CH, et al. A step-up approach or open necrosectomy for necrotizing pancreatitis. N Engl J Med. 2010;362(16):1491-502.
12. Asbun HJ, Moekotte AL, Vissers FL, Kunzler F, Cipriani F, Alseidi A, et al. The Miami International evidence-based guidelines on minimally invasive pancreas resection. Ann Surg. 2020;271(1):1-14.
13. van Hilst J, de Rooij T, Bosscha K, Brinkman DJ, van Dieren S, Dijkgraaf MG, et al. Laparoscopic versus open pancreatoduodenectomy for pancreatic or periampullary tumours (LEOPARD-2): a multicentre, patient-blinded, randomised controlled phase 2/3 trial. Lancet Gastroenterol Hepatol. 2019;4(3):199-207.
14. Riviere D, Gurusamy KS, Kooby DA, Vollmer CM, Besselink MGH, Davidson BR, et al. Laparoscopic versus open distal pancreatectomy for pancreatic cancer. Cochrane Database Syst Rev. 2016;4:CD011391.
15. de Rooij T, van Hilst J, Vogel JA, van Santvoort HC, de Boer MT, Boerma D, et al. Minimally invasive versus open distal pancreatectomy (LEOPARD): study protocol for a randomized controlled trial. Trials. 2017;18(1):166.

16. Palanivelu C, Senthilnathan P, Sabnis SC, Babu NS, Gurumurthy SS, Vijai NA, et al. Randomized clinical trial of laparoscopic versus open pancreatoduodenectomy for periampullary tumours. Br J Surg. 2017;104(11):1443-50.
17. Barreto S. Pancreatic cancer. In: Barreto SG, Windsor JA (eds). Surgery of the Pancreas and Biliary Tree. Singapore: Springer Nature; 2018.
18. Shrikhande S, Barreto S, Sirohi B, Bal M, Shrimali RK, Chacko RT, et al. Indian Council of Medical Research Consensus document for the management of pancreatic cancer. Indian J Med Paediatr Oncol. 2019;40(1):9-14.
19. Hariharan D, Constantinides VA, Froeling FE, Tekkis PP, Kocher HM. The role of laparoscopy and laparoscopic ultrasound in the preoperative staging of pancreatico-biliary cancers--A meta-analysis. Eur J Surg Oncol. 2010;36(10):941-8.
20. Society of American Gastrointestinal and Endoscopic Surgeons. Guidelines for Diagnostic Laparoscopy. [online] Available from: http://www.sages.org/publications/guidelines/guidelines-for-diagnostic-laparoscopy/ accessed July 8th, 2016. [Last accessed November 2021].
21. Levy J, Tahiri M, Vanounou T, Maimon G, Bergman S. Diagnostic laparoscopy with ultrasound still has a role in the staging of pancreatic cancer: a systematic review of the literature. HPB Surg. 2016;2016:8092109.
22. Liu R, Wakabayashi G, Palanivelu C, Tsung A, Yang K, Goh BKP, et al. International consensus statement on robotic pancreatic surgery. Hepatobiliary Surg Nutr. 2019;8(4):345-60.
23. Conlon KC, de Rooij T, van Hilst J, Abu-Hidal M, Fleshman J, Talamonti M, et al. Minimally invasive pancreatic resections: cost and value perspectives. HPB (Oxford). 2017;19(3):225-33.
24. Chaudhary A, Barreto S, Talole S, Singh A, Perwaiz A, Singh T. Early discharge after Pancreatoduodenectomy - what helps and what prevents? Pancreas. 2015;44:273-8.
25. Cao Y, Gu HY, Huang ZD, Wu YP, Zhang Q, Luo J, et al. Impact of enhanced recovery after surgery on postoperative recovery for pancreaticoduodenectomy: pooled analysis of observational study. Front Oncol. 2019;9:687.
26. Gurusamy KS, Riviere D, van Laarhoven CJH, Besselink M, Abu-Hilal M, Davidson BR, et al. Cost-effectiveness of laparoscopic versus open distal pancreatectomy for pancreatic cancer. PLoS One. 2017;12(12):e0189631.
27. Magge DR, Zenati MS, Hamad A, Rieser C, Zureikat AH, Zeh HJ, et al. Comprehensive comparative analysis of cost-effectiveness and perioperative outcomes between open, laparoscopic, and robotic distal pancreatectomy. HPB (Oxford). 2018;20(12):1172-80.
28. Moekotte AL, Rawashdeh A, Asbun HJ, Coimbra FJ, Edil BH, Jarufe N, et al. Safe implementation of minimally invasive pancreas resection: a systematic review. HPB (Oxford). 2020;22(5):637-48.
29. de Rooij T, Cipriani F, Rawashdeh M, van Dieren S, Barbaro S, Abuawwad M, et al. Single-surgeon learning curve in 111 laparoscopic distal pancreatectomies: does operative time tell the whole story? J Am Coll Surg. 2017;224(5):826-32e1.
30. Choi M, Hwang HK, Lee WJ, Kang CM. Total laparoscopic pancreatico-duodenectomy in patients with periampullary tumors: a learning curve analysis. Surg Endosc. 2021;35(6):2636-44.

31. Shakir M, Boone BA, Polanco PM, Zenati MS, Hogg ME, Tsung A, et al. The learning curve for robotic distal pancreatectomy: an analysis of outcomes of the first 100 consecutive cases at a high-volume pancreatic centre. HPB (Oxford). 2015;17(7):580-6.
32. van Hilst J, de Rooij T, Hilal MA, Asbun HJ, Barkun J, Boggi U, et al. Worldwide survey on opinions and use of minimally invasive pancreatic resection. HPB (Oxford). 2017;19(3):190-204.
33. Nickel F, Haney CM, Kowalewski KF, Probst P, Limen EF, Kalkum E, et al. Laparoscopic versus open pancreaticoduodenectomy: a systematic review and meta-analysis of randomized controlled trials. Ann Surg. 2020;271(1):54-66.
34. Sun YM, Wang Y, Mao YX, Wang W. The safety and feasibility of enhanced recovery after surgery in patients undergoing pancreaticoduodenectomy: an updated meta-analysis. Biomed Res Int. 2020;2020:7401276.
35. Doctor N, Hussain M, Barreto S. Delayed single stage necrosectomy for infected pancreatic necrosis. HPB (Oxford). 2008;10:122.
36. Shrikhande S, Barreto S, Somashekar B, Suradkar K, Shetty GS, Talole S, et al. Evolution of pancreatoduodenectomy in a tertiary cancer centre in India: improved results from service reconfiguration. Pancreatology. 2013;13:63-71.
37. Bassi C, Marchegiani G, Dervenis C, Sarr M, Hilal MA, Adham M, et al. The 2016 update of the International Study Group (ISGPS) definition and grading of postoperative pancreatic fistula: 11 years after. Surgery. 2017;161(3):584-91.
38. Wente MN, Bassi C, Dervenis C, Fingerhut A, Gouma DJ, Izbicki JR, et al. Delayed gastric emptying (DGE) after pancreatic surgery: a suggested definition by the International Study Group of Pancreatic Surgery (ISGPS). Surgery. 2007;142(5):761-8.
39. Wente MN, Veit JA, Bassi C, Dervenis C, Fingerhut A, Gouma DJ, et al. Postpancreatectomy hemorrhage (PPH): an International Study Group of Pancreatic Surgery (ISGPS) definition. Surgery. 2007;142(1):20-5.
40. Petrov MS, Shanbhag S, Chakraborty M, Phillips ARJ, Windsor JA. Organ failure and infection of pancreatic necrosis as determinants of mortality in patients with acute pancreatitis. Gastroenterology. 2010;139(3):813-20.

CHAPTER

Laparoscopic Pancreaticoduodenectomy

Siddhartha Mishra, Rajesh Bhojwani

■ INTRODUCTION

Ever since the popularization of pancreatoduodenectomy (PD) as the only curative option for pancreatic and periampullary malignancy in 1935 by Whipple, it continues to be high on the list amongst the most complicated abdominal operations. Over the period, as the techniques of performing this surgery have improved and with the introduction of electrosurgical devices, there has been a significant improvement in the morbidity and mortality rates associated with this surgery, and survival rates up to 30% have been achieved in resectable patients.[1]

The possibility of exploring the advantages of minimal access surgery in improving the outcome of this surgery was first envisaged by Gagner and Pomp in 1994 in a case of pancreatic divisum.[2] Despite the introduction of laparoscopic pancreatoduodenectomy (LPD) almost three decades back, it continues to be a formidable challenge and a highly specialized procedure. According to a large, nationwide, American database, only <5% of hepatobiliopancreatic procedures were reported to be carried out by a minimally invasive approach.[3] The reason for this is the retroperitoneal location of this organ along with its proximity to major vessels.[4] The daunting task of performing three anastomosis requires considerable expertise and a long learning curve. As surgeons become more adept in advanced laparoscopy, there is increasing evidence demonstrating not only the safety and feasibility of laparoscopic pancreatic resection, but also potential advantages in postoperative recovery and equivalent oncological outcome.[5] Researchers have confirmed the utility of MIS in decreasing the proinflammatory and immunologic response to surgical trauma that is often associated with a superior oncologic result.[6,7] Nevertheless, LPD has failed to reach a sufficient level of evidence-based efficacy to enable a routine application.[8]

In general, there are two approaches to minimally invasive pancreaticoduodenectomy (MIPD): A total laparoscopic approach where the anastomoses (pancreaticojejunostomy, hepaticojejunostomy, and gastrojejunostomy) along with the resection are done intracorporeally, and the laparoscopic-assisted or hybrid approach, where reconstruction is done through a small incision which is also used for specimen extraction. Studies have shown equivalent outcomes for both of these procedures.[9]

Whatever be the approach, a technique based on precise dissection planes, meticulous hemostasis, delicate handling of vascular structures, wide lymphadenectomy, contamination avoidance, and minimization of excessive incisional trauma is universally beneficial to all patients undergoing pancreatectomy by any method.[10] These are also the basic tenets of a successful minimally invasive PD.

■ INDICATIONS

There is still no consensus regarding the suitability of patients for LPD and it is often guided by the expertise and learning curve of the treating team. Periampullary lesions are often considered ideal for LPD because of their localized nature and absence of major vessel involvement.[11] Ampullary lesions tend to present early with jaundice and have dilated biliary and pancreatic duct, which make anastomosis easier and reduces the chances of leak. Pancreatic head tumors less than 3 cm and lower common bile duct (CBD) lesions without extrabiliary involvement are also good candidates for LPD.[12]

Low-grade malignancies such as mucinous cystic neoplasms, intraductal papillary mucinous neoplasm (IPMN), and neuroendocrine tumor (NET) are also considered ideal because of the lack of nodal and vascular involvement in these lesions.[13]

Besides the established contraindications of laparoscopic procedures, the contraindications for LPD include patients who require concomitant vessel reconstruction or anatomical hepatectomy.[13] In general, LPD may be technically very difficult in patients with severe obesity, cholangitis, pancreatitis, and potential risk of combined major vascular resection.[14] Particularly when dealing with mid-bile duct cancer, problems with resection-margin status may be encountered during the operation, which make LPD more difficult.[14] Patients with a suspected pancreatic head mass lesion in the setting of chronic pancreatitis are also poor candidates for LPD because of the obliteration of tissue planes due to chronic inflammation.[12] Patients with comorbidities and those in poor performance status who cannot tolerate pneumoperitoneum for a prolonged duration may not be suitable to undergo LPD.[14]

Intraoperatively, wise decision-making for conversion to laparotomy is paramount. For patient safety, failure to progress within 1 hour of dissection as a result of severe pancreatitis or adhesions, unexpected vascular invasion, unexpected adjacent organ involvement requiring combined organ resection, unusual vascular anatomy, and uncontrolled bleeding may warrant conversion to laparotomy.[14]

■ OPERATIVE STEPS (AUTHOR'S TECHNIQUE)

Slow adoption of LPD worldwide is predominant because of the absence of standardization of operative steps. Surgeons modify and adopt techniques in accordance with their experience and this heterogeneity amongst pancreatic surgeons is one of the reasons for the slow percolation and wide adoption of this technique. In general, LPD consists of the "Resection" and the "Reconstruction."

Resection

The operation is started with five ports in the upper abdomen. The camera port is inserted at the infraumbilical position. An arc is formed in the form of an inverted bucket-handle with the two ends at the right and left subcostal positions. These two ends are used for insertion of two ports, one 10–12 mm on the left subcostal region for the surgeon's right hand and one 5 mm for the assistant to retract the gallbladder. The remaining two ports (both 10–12 mm) are inserted midway on the arc. The surgeon stands on the left side of the patient and starts with dissection at the porta hepatis, while the gallbladder fundus is grasped to provide retraction by the assistant. The gastroduodenal artery is ligated and divided as the first step. This is then followed by tracing the right hepatic artery till its confirmed course toward the right side. Cystic artery is then identified and divided. This opens up the Calot triangle which allows passage of a vascular sling from left to the right side. After confirmation, the CBD is divided, having procured a sample for bile culture. The hepatic side of the divided CBD is then secured with a bulldog clamp and the specimen side with a suture. The dissection at the porta is then followed retrogradely to dissect the CBD and the tissue and lymphatics and lymph nodes away from the portal vein which is laid bared. With the help of a gold finger, a retropancreatic tunnel is then secured halfway through from the top. Gastrocolic momentum is divided, right gastroepiploic vessels secured, and the duodenum divided beyond the pylorus with a stapler. The next step is to Kocherize the duodenum from first to the second part and also from the third to the second part till the left renal vein is seen and the pancreas and duodenum have been lifted up from the inferior vena cava (IVC). The dissection then shifts to the infracolic compartment and the jejunum is divided with a stapler app 3 inches away from the DJ. The mesojejunum is then divided with ultrascission and the divided jejunum taken to the right side from behind the mesentery.

The surgeon now changes his position and starts operating from between the legs of the patient. This aligns the ergonomics and gives him a straight field to operate upon. The middle colic vein is then followed to identify the portal vein and the retropancreatic tunnel is secured from below upward. The complete tunnel is secured, and the pancreatic neck divided with ultrascission. An infant feeding tube is now used to identify and cannulate the pancreatic duct. With the vertical alignment of the portal vein and divided neck of pancreas, the specimen now hangs only with the gallbladder and the uncinate process. Having confirmed the availability of hemlock clips of various sizes, metal clips, ultrascission function, suction function, and 5-0 prolene sutures, the uncinate is now dissected with serial dissection, identification of vessels, securement with clips, and ultrascission. Care is taken to conclusively clip the inferior pancreaticoduodenal vein, superior pancreaticoduodenal vein, and conclusively avoid inadvertent injury to aberrant right hepatic artery arising from the superior mesenteric artery and the first jejunal vein. Complete vision of the uncinate process from the superior mesenteric vessels now allows the specimen to hang only on the gallbladder—the specimen is flipped over the liver and the field retracted with the gallbladder attached to provide a wide exposure for reconstruction.

Reconstruction

The pancreaticojejunostomy is undertaken first with a surgeon in the same position. We prefer a duct to mucosa technique. The outer layer is done with 2-0 silk and the ductal sutures with 4-0 PDS around an infant feeding tube which keeps the lumen of a small pancreatic duct open and enables proper entry and exit points of the needle. It also serves as a stent (not fixed) which serves only to facilitate the anastomosis. Thereafter, the surgeon moves to the left of the patient and hepaticojejunostomy is performed with 4-0 interrupted sutures with the same jejunal loop app. 10 cm proximal to the pancreatic anastomosis.

Gallbladder is now taken off its bed and the specimen is inserted in a retrieval bag. At this juncture, a small incision is made in the midline epigastric region ($\approx$5–6 cm) through which the specimen is withdrawn and gastrojejunostomy and jejunojejunostomy fashioned. For a young patient who is cosmetically conscious, gastrojejunostomy and jejunojejunostomy are also fashioned intracorporeally with staplers and the specimen is withdrawn through a suprapubic incision. Two drains are inserted, and the nasogastric tube is advanced into the efferent limb.

Intraoperative Pictures Depicting the Procedure

Figures 1 to 10 depicting the intraoperative procedure of laparoscopic pancreaticoduodenectomy.

LAPAROSCOPIC VERSUS OPEN PANCREATICODUODENECTOMY

Ever since the introduction of LPD, a large number of retrospective studies have been published comparing its perioperative, postoperative, and oncological outcomes against open PD. These studies have confirmed that the traditional benefits of laparoscopic procedures such as less postoperative pain, faster recovery, and equivalent oncological outcomes are applicable even for the patients undergoing LPD, however, at the cost of a longer operative time.

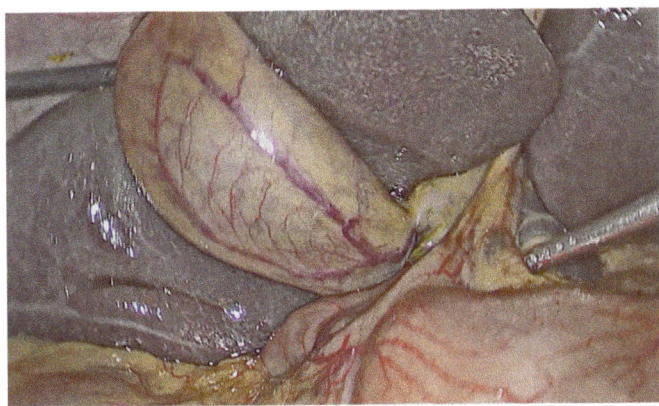

Fig. 1: Field retraction with the gallbladder and a suture hitching the ligamentum teres to the anterior.

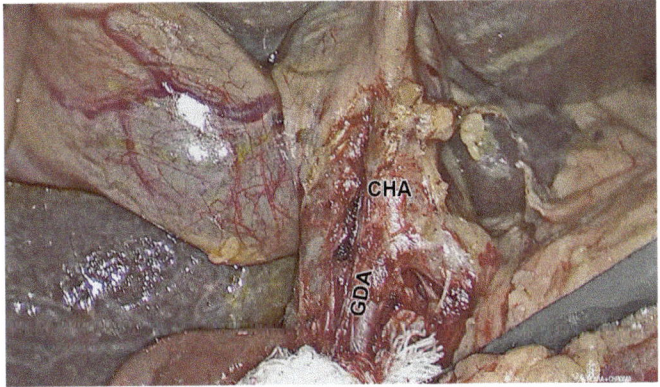

Fig. 2: Common hepatic artery (CHA) and gastroduodenal artery (GDA).

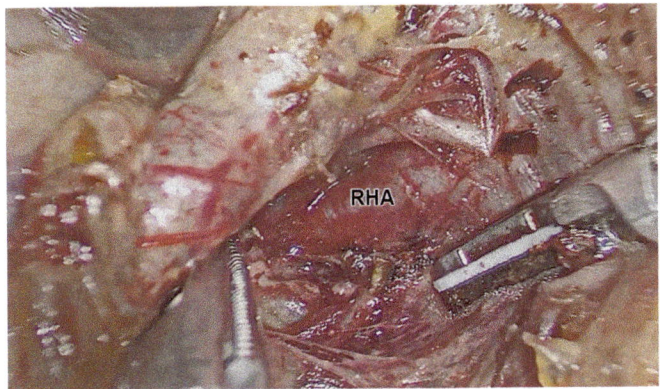

Fig. 3: Right hepatic artery (RHA) seen behind the common bile duct.

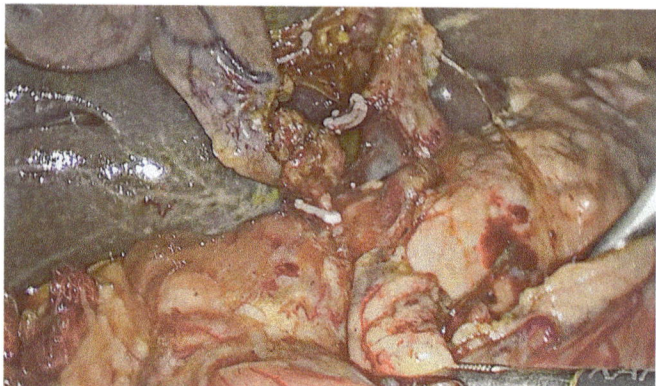

Fig. 4: Common bile duct and gastroduodenal artery divided and portal vein dissection.

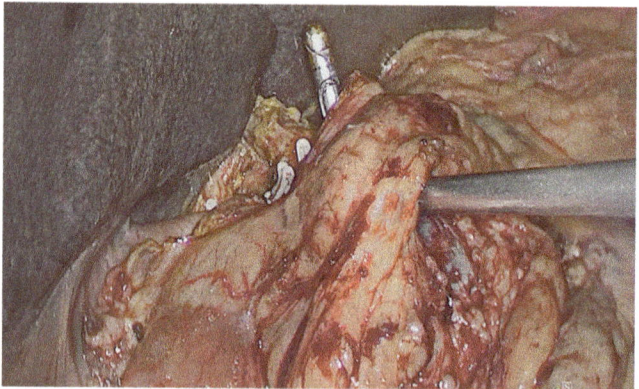

Fig. 5: Tunnel created behind the pancreatic neck.

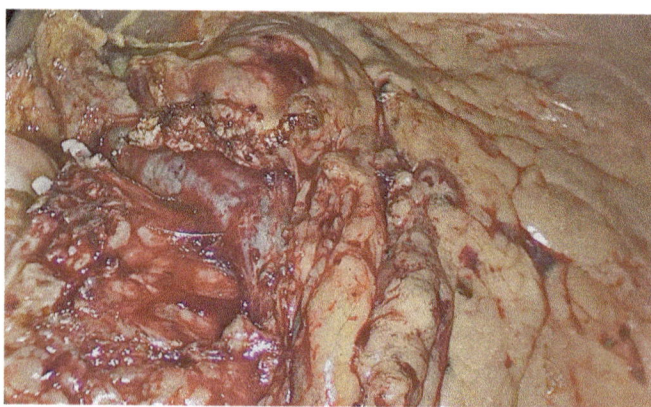

Fig. 6: Pancreatic neck transected.

Laparoscopic Pancreaticoduodenectomy

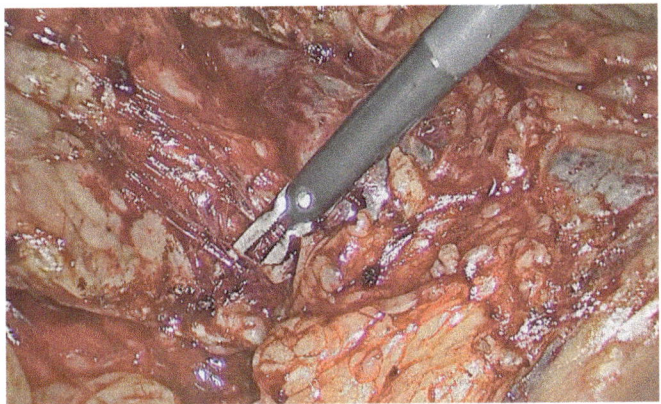

Fig. 7: Uncinate dissection.

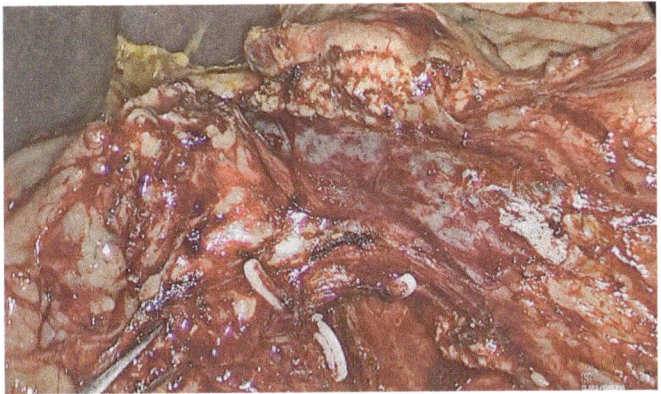

Fig. 8: Completion of uncinate dissection.

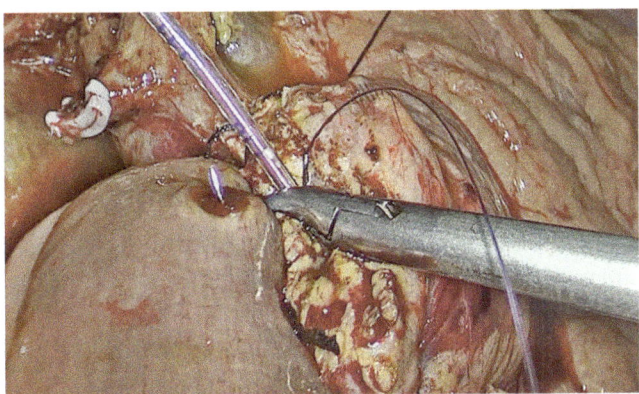

Fig. 9: Pancreaticojejunal duct to mucosa anastomosis. Infant feeding tube is kept as pancreatic stent.

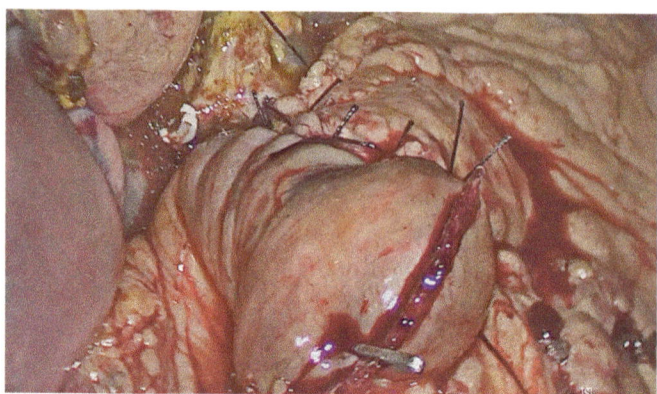

Fig. 10: Completed pancreaticojejunal anastomosis.

Meng et al. found that compared with patients who underwent open PD, patients who underwent LPD had a shorter time to first passage of flatus and oral intake, while no differences were seen in blood loss, length of intensive care unit (ICU) stay, node positivity, or R0 resection between the laparoscopic and open groups, with no significant differences in major complications including the rate of postoperative pancreatic fistula.[15]

Asbun and Stauffer compared the outcomes based on morbidity and mortality and found shorted ICU and hospital stay, lower blood loss and transfusions, and a higher retrieval of lymph nodes. Although operative time was statistically longer for LPD, there was no difference in overall complications and pancreatic fistula rate between LPD and open PD. They inferred that LPD is safe and feasible and the outcomes are better than open PD.[16]

Croome et al. analyzed and found that after operation, the open PD group stayed longer in the hospital (average: 9 days) compared to the LPD group (average: 6 days). Moreover, progression-free survival was longer in LPD compared to the open PD group. In patients administered with adjuvant chemotherapy, median time until commencement of treatment was also shorter in LPD (48 days, ranging from 17 to 116 days) compared to open PD (59 days, ranging from 25 to 302 days) and a significantly smaller proportion of patients in the LPD group had a delay of >56 days. Intraoperative transfusions and delayed gastric emptying occurred less frequently in the LPD group. In terms of overall survival, there was no significant difference between the two. Based on these results, authors emphasized that the LPD was not only feasible but also had significant advantages over the traditional open approach.[17] Similar results have been reflected in the study by Jacobs et al. in 2013.[18]

A large meta-analysis was published by Zhang et al. in 2019 based on two randomized controlled trials (RCTs) and 26 retrospective comparative studies of LPD and open PD, preliminarily confirmed the feasibility and potential advantages of LPD; among 39,771 patients, including 3,543 in the LPD group and the remaining 36,228 in the open PD group. There were no significant differences between the two groups in terms of the major morbidity, mortality, re-operation, and 90-day readmission rates. LPD was associated with less blood loss, lower blood transfusion rate, lower incidence of overall postoperative complications, shorter length of ICU stay and length of stay (LOS), more harvested lymph nodes, and higher R0 resection rate than open PD. However, LPD was associated with a longer operative time and a smaller tumor size.[19]

Despite a large number of studies promoting LPD for its purported benefits, there have been studies that question the application of laparoscopic techniques in managing malignant lesions.[20,21] All these reports pose challenges to the preoperative and long-term survival outcomes of patients with minimally invasive operations for all malignant tumors including LPD. A recent study from the National Cancer Data Base (NCDB) from the American College of Surgeons and the American Cancer Society reports an unacceptably high mortality rate for the laparoscopic approach compared with the open PD.[22]

Dokmak et al. in his retrospective comparative study found that patients in the LPD group had a lower body mass index (BMI), a softer pancreas, longer operating time (342 vs. 264 minutes; $p < 0.001$), more grade C pancreatic fistula (24 vs. 6%; $p = 0.007$), bleedings (24 vs. 7%; $p = 0.02$), and revision surgery (24 vs. 11%; $p = 0.09$). According to these results, the authors concluded that LPD was not to be recommended on a routine basis.[23]

Similarly Corcione et al. found that LPD does not provide significant benefits compared to the open approach but may do so, in specialized centers with surgeons who have acquired highly advanced skills in LPD. He stressed on the importance of learning curve in influencing the overall outcome of LPD.[24]

It is worthwhile to mention that there is a lot of selection and institutional biases in these studies. Surgeons in their initial phase of their learning curve tend to choose patients with smaller tumors, without nodal, vascular, or hepatic involvement. These factors can influence the overall outcome in these patients to a great extent and have to be taken into consideration before reaching any conclusion regarding the safety and efficacy of LPD.

RANDOMIZED CONTROLLED TRIALS ON LAPAROSCOPIC PANCREATODUODENECTOMY

Almost all authors in previous studies concluded that there was a need for high-quality RCTs to reduce the probability of selection bias in these studies. Recently, a randomized LEOPARD-2 trial was initiated with the aim to compare time to functional recovery after laparoscopic versus open PD.[25] The LEOPARD-2 trial was a multicenter, patient-blinded, parallel-group, randomized controlled phase 2/3 superiority trial comparing laparoscopic with open PD with each participating centers performing at least 20 LPDs annually. LPD did not reduce time to functional recovery and that postoperative complications, costs, and quality of life were comparable. These findings were in contrast with the single-center PLOT and PADULAP randomized trials, which both showed shorter length of hospital stay after laparoscopic than after open PD (7 vs. 13 days in 64 patients and 14 vs. 17 days in 66 patients).[26,27] In these trials, postoperative morbidity and mortality were lower or similar after laparoscopic versus open PD. The conversion rate was 3% (1 of 32 patients) in the PLOT trial and 5% (8 of 34 patients) in the PADULAP trial. The LEOPARD-2 trial was prematurely terminated because of safety concerns related to higher 90-day complication-related mortality in the laparoscopic group.

Meta-analysis published in 2019 included the three RCTs (PLOT, PADULAP and LEOPARD-2 trails) with a total of 224 patients.[28] PLOT trial only included patients with periampullary cancers, while the LEOPARD-2 trial and the PADULAP trial included patients with benign and malignant conditions. Performance and detection bias in both PLOT and the PADULAP trials revealed a high risk of bias score as they performed no blinding. The LEOPARD-2 trial received a low risk of bias score for patient blinding as these were blinded with the help of a large abdominal dressing.

Results of this meta-analysis showed that there was no significant difference in postoperative pancreatic fistula (POPF) and post-pancreatectomy hemorrhage (PPH) grades B and C and between the two groups. All reports of delayed gastric emptying were pooled and there was no significant difference between the two groups. Bile leak showed no significant difference. There was significantly less blood loss in the LPD group. There were no significant differences in the reoperation rates between the two groups. Also, there was no difference in the R0 resection rates between the two groups. All trials reported the number of lymph nodes harvested (212 participants). There was no significant difference between the two groups in terms of nodes harvested. Duration of operation was reported by all trials (224 patients) and it was significantly higher in the LPD group.

The meta-analysis concluded that with the current level of evidence, the two procedures cannot be considered equivalent. While two trials originally measured significantly shorter LOS in the LPD group, the multicentric LEOPARD-2 trial offered nonsignificant opposing results with longer LOS in the LPD group. After meta-analysis, the pooled results were still in favor of the LPD group, however, not significantly.

On reviewing the surgery videos of participating surgeons in LEOPARD-2 trial, at least 20% of the surgeons were rated as "below average" in their surgical skills. This trial showed that including an adequate credentialing system into the trial design and upholding a high quality of surgical performance by training, mentoring, and proctoring are important factors to adequately evaluate new surgical techniques.

CONCLUSION

The advantage of minimal access in influencing the outcome of surgery is a well-established fact, however, implementing it in a technically intricate procedure such as pancreaticoduodenectomy has its own challenges. Studies have proved its noninferiority over OPD in terms of oncological and perioperative outcomes, however, there are no RCTs available which compare the long-term survival advantages of this procedure. LEOPARD-2 trial has raised some serious safety concerns about this procedure. We must be mindful of the extent that the skill of the surgeon has on the outcome of the operation and the differing abilities of surgeons to learn at different stages of the learning curve. Therefore, a possible avenue to achieve this would be using surgical simulation machines to assess how different instructional methods affect blood loss and trauma incurred in subsequent simulated operations. We must pay attention to the patient's actual situation and combine the different surgical methods reasonably, in order to optimize patient outcomes and mitigate unnecessary healthcare expenditures. This aspect is especially relevant for patients from our region where the healthcare cost is a major stumbling block.

OUR EXPERIENCE

Authors performed the first laparoscopic-assisted pancreaticoduodenectomy in the year 2010. Thereafter, the pace was slow for a few years and only seven laparoscopic-assisted resections were performed in the next 5 years with one re-exploration for an intra-abdominal bleed. The procedure gathered pace in the last 5 years, and we have now performed 31 LPDs, out of a total of 496 PDs (2002–2018) in our department. A detailed analysis is being done to come up with a formal publication.

REFERENCES

1. Strobel O, Neoptolemos J, Jaeger D, Buechler MW. Optimizing the outcomes of pancreatic cancer surgery. Nat Rev Clin Oncol. 2019;16(1):11-26.
2. Gagner M, Pomp A. Laparoscopic pylorus-preserving pancreatoduodenectomy. Surg Endosc. 1994;8(5):408-10.
3. Ejaz A, Sachs T, He J, Spolverato G, Hirose K, Ahuja N, et al. A comparison of open and minimally invasive surgery for hepatic and pancreatic resections using the Nationwide Inpatient Sample. Surg. 2014;156(3):538-47.
4. Liu M, Ji S, Xu W, Liu W, Qin Y, Hu Q, et al. Laparoscopic pancreaticoduodenectomy: are the best times coming? World J Surg Oncol. 2019;17:81.

5. Torphy RJ, Friedman C, Halpern A, Chapman BC, Ahrendt SS, McCarter MM, et al. Comparing short-term and oncologic outcomes of minimally invasive versus open pancreaticoduodenectomy across low and high volume centers. Ann Surg. 2019;270(6):1147-55.
6. Goldfarb M, Brower S, Schwaitzberg SD. Minimally invasive surgery and cancer: controversies part 1. Surg Endosc. 2010;24(2):304-34.
7. Sharma B, Baxter N, Grantcharov T. Outcomes after laparoscopic techniques in major gastrointestinal surgery. Curr Opin Crit Care. 2010;16(4):371-6.
8. Bencini L, Annecchiarico M, Farsi M, Bartolini I, Mirasolo V, Guerra F, et al. Minimally invasive surgical approach to pancreatic malignancies. World J Gastro Oncol. 2015;7(12):411-21.
9. Dulucq JL, Wintringer P, Stabilini C, Feryn T, Perissat J, Mahajna A. Are major laparoscopic pancreatic resections worthwhile? A prospective study of 32 patients in a single institution. Surg Endosc Interventional Techniques. 2005;19(8):1028-34.
10. Stauffer JA, Asbun HJ. Minimally invasive pancreatic resectional techniques' William R. Jarnagin; Blumgart's Surgery of the Liver, Biliary Tract, and Pancreas. Philadelphia: Elsevier; 2017. pp. 1028-30.
11. Liang S, Hameed U, Jayaraman S. Laparoscopic pancreatectomy: indications and outcomes. World J Gastroenterol. 2014;20(39):14246-54.
12. Palanivelu C, Jani K, Senthilnathan P, Parthasarathi R, Rajapandian S, Madhankumar MV. Laparoscopic pancreaticoduodenectomy: technique and outcomes. J Am Coll Surgeons. 2007;205(2):222-30.
13. Umemura A, Nitta H, Takahara T, Hasegawa Y, Sasaki A. Current status of laparoscopic pancreaticoduodenectomy and pancreatectomy. Asian J Surg. 2018;41(2):106-14.
14. Navarro JG, Kang CM. Pitfalls for laparoscopic pancreaticoduodenectomy: need for a stepwise approach. Ann Gastroenterol Surg. 2019;3(3):254-68.
15. Meng LW, Cai YQ, Li YB, Cai H, Peng B. Comparison of laparoscopic and open pancreaticoduodenectomy for the treatment of nonpancreatic periampullary adenocarcinomas. Surg Laparosc Endosc Percutan Tech. 2018;28(1):56-61.
16. Asbun HJ, Stauffer JA. Laparoscopic vs open pancreaticoduodenectomy: overall outcomes and severity of complications using the Accordion Severity Grading System. J Am Coll Surgeons. 2012;215(6):810-9.
17. Croome KP, Farnell MB, Que FG, et al. Pancreaticoduodenectomy with major vascular resection: a comparison of laparoscopic versus open approaches. J Gastroint Surg. 2015;19(1):189-94.
18. Jacobs MJ, Kamyab A. Total laparoscopic pancreaticoduodenectomy. JSLS: J Soc Laproend. 2013;17(2):188.
19. Zhang H, Lan X, Peng B, Li B. Is total laparoscopic pancreaticoduodenectomy superior to open procedure? A meta-analysis. World J Gastroenterol. 2019;25(37):5711-31.
20. Ramirez PT, Frumovitz M, Pareja R, Lopez A, Vieira M, Ribeiro R, et al. Minimally invasive versus abdominal radical hysterectomy for cervical cancer. N Engl J Med. 2018;379(20):1895-904.
21. Melamed A, Margul DJ, Chen L, Keating NL, Del Carmen MG, Yang J, et al. Survival after minimally invasive radical hysterectomy for early-stage cervical cancer. N Engl J Med. 2018;379(20):1905-14.

22. Sharpe SM, Talamonti MS, Wang CE, Prinz RA, Roggin KK, Bentrem DJ, et al. Early national experience with laparoscopic pancreaticoduodenectomy for ductal adenocarcinoma: a comparison of laparoscopic pancreaticoduodenectomy and open pancreaticoduodenectomy from the National Cancer Data Base. J Am Coll Surgeons. 2015;221(1):175-84.
23. Dokmak S, Ftériche FS, Aussilhou B, Bensafta Y, Lévy P, Ruszniewski P, et al. Laparoscopic pancreaticoduodenectomy should not be routine for resection of periampullary tumors. J Am Coll Surgeons. 2015;220(5):831-8.
24. Corcione F, Pirozzi F, Cuccurullo D, Piccolboni D, Caracino V, Galante F, et al. Laparoscopic pancreaticoduodenectomy: experience of 22 cases. Surg Endosc. 2013;27(6):2131-6.
25. van Hilst J, de Rooij T, Bosscha K, Brinkman DJ, van Dieren S, Dijkgraaf MG, et al. Laparoscopic versus open pancreatoduodenectomy for pancreatic or periampullary tumours (LEOPARD-2): a multicentre, patient-blinded, randomised controlled phase 2/3 trial. Lancet Gastroenterol. 2019;4(3):199-207.
26. Palanisamy S. Pancreatic Head and Peri-ampullary Cancer Laparoscopic vs Open Surgical Treatment Trial (PLOT) (NCT02081131); 2014. [online] Available from: https://clinicaltrials.gov/ct2/show/NCT02081131. [Last accessed November 2021].
27. Poves I. PADULAP Study: To compare postoperative and pathologic results between open and laparoscopic approach for pancreaticoduodenectomy (ISRCTN93168938); 2013. [online] Available from: http://isrctn.com/ISRCTN93168938. [Last accessed November 2021].
28. Nickel F, Haney CM, Kowalewski KF, Probst P, Limen EF, Kalkum E, et al. Laparoscopic versus open pancreaticoduodenectomy: a systematic review and meta-analysis of randomized controlled trials. Ann Surg. 2020;271(1):54-66.

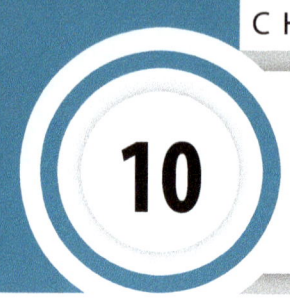

CHAPTER 10

Initiating Robotic Pancreaticoduodenectomy

Ruchit H Kansaria, Manish S Bhandare, Vikram Chaudhari,
Ammiel Arra, Shailesh V Shrikhande

■ INTRODUCTION

Since its inception by Walter Kausch in 1909 and subsequent popularization by Allen Whipple in the 1930s, pancreaticoduodenectomy (PD) has been one of the most intimidating procedures in surgery. Significant morbidity and mortality associated with this procedure had placed its role into question, in the earlier times. Due to standardization of the operative techniques, newer surgical devices, advancements in the field of anesthesia, better perioperative care as well as effective management of complications, have greatly minimized the risks of adverse postoperative clinical events.

While the basic aspects of resection and reconstruction have remained relatively constant, several modifications have been proposed in an attempt to minimize the risk of complications. Among these include the pylorus-preserving PD in 1978 by Traverso and Longmire, which attempted to minimize the incidence and severity of postgastrectomy syndromes.[1] To reduce postoperative pancreatic fistula (POPF), multiple variations in pancreaticojejunostomy (PJ) and pancreaticogastrostomy have been described. Standardization of anastomotic technique helps reduce postoperative pancreatic fistula-induced morbidity, and no single technique has shown clear superiority over the other.[2]

Cameron et al. at Johns Hopkins would eventually outline a morbidity of 30–40% and mortality of 1–3%, which is currently the proposed standard for high-volume centers internationally.[3]

At out center, we have a dedicated pancreatic unit working together as a multidisciplinary team, which has led to improvement in morbidity and mortality after major PD. From 2012 to 2017, we have had morbidity rate of 30% and a mortality rate of 2.8%.[4] We have gradually incorporated neoadjuvant protocols for borderline resectable disease, superior mesenteric artery (SMA) first approach, and also routinely perform multivisceral and vascular resections. We believe the improvement in overall outcomes observed in our patients has been possible due to sustained and continuous efforts toward achieving excellence in all aspects of pancreatic cancer care that begins with quality of surgery and perioperative care.

Although majority of cases in our series are by open approach, our experience with minimally invasive pancreaticoduodenectomy (MIPD) continues to evolve with current focus on patient selection and standardization of the surgical steps.

The first laparoscopic PD was performed by Gagner and Pomp in 1994.[5] Laparoscopic techniques are firmly established approaches for various benign and malignant diseases, but the difficulties encountered in its implementation for PD has limited its widespread use. Feasibility by a few extremely skilled surgeons in high-volume centers does not make minimal access surgery in case of PD as the standard of care. After adequate navigation of the learning curve, it should be possible for most surgeons to perform a safe and competent surgery. It needs adequately powered randomized trials demonstrating its equivalence to the open approach in terms of perioperative outcomes, oncological adequacy, and long-term survival. The reluctance in acceptance of laparoscopic pancreaticoduodenectomy (LPD) has been attributed to several inherent limitations of laparoscopy (limited range of instrument motion, reduced fine motor control, poor ergonomics, two-dimensional vision), which seem to be amplified when attempting to perform precise dissection and reconstruction. The most difficult aspects of PD include uncinate dissection and pancreaticojejunal anastomosis.

With the advent of robotic surgery, many of the deficiencies of laparoscopic surgery have been overcome by technological advancements, allowing for superior magnification, greater range of movement (endowrist), extremely precise dissection, tremor filtration, and improved ergonomics. The learning curve for robotic pancreaticoduodenectomy (RPD) compared to laparoscopic pancreaticoduodenectomy (LPD) is less arduous and hence has led to a greater acceptability amongst surgeons. In 2003, Giulianotti et al. published a case series verifying the feasibility of robotic pancreatectomy; the series included eight robot-assisted pancreaticoduodenectomy (RAPD) and five robot-assisted distal pancreatectomy (RADP) cases.[6] We have done 83 minimal invasive PDs, which include 8 total robotic, 3 total laparoscopic, 8 laparoscopic resections with robotic reconstruction, 43 laparoscopic resections with open reconstruction, and 21 robotic resections with open reconstruction. We ensured patient safety by staggering our approach initially, by standardizing resections first before embarking upon reconstructions. We believe that this approach is optimally suited to those teams which are planning to get into minimally access pancreatic surgery. We will describe our approach to patients being planned for robotic PD.

TECHNICAL ASPECTS

Selection Criteria for Minimally Invasive Pancreaticoduodenectomy

- In order to ensure good perioperative outcomes and adequate oncological clearance, it is prudent to be judicious and highly selective in offering the

robotic approach to the individual patients, especially in the initial phase of the learning curve.
- Indications for robotic PD at our institute include:
  - Patients with duodenal, ampullary carcinoma, early distal cholangiocarcinoma, or clearly resectable pancreatic carcinoma
  - No features of borderline resectability on preoperative imaging
  - Body mass index (BMI) of <28
  - No previous history of cholangitis or multiple biliary stent exchanges
  - Patients with no previous major upper abdominal surgery
  - Minimally invasive pancreaticoduodenectomy (MIPD) usually requires longer operative times, hence younger patients with good cardiopulmonary reserve, ASA I and ASA II (American Society of Anesthesiologists) are preferred
  - Patients with low risk of POPF with dilated pancreatic and biliary duct are preferred.

Preoperative Workup

- Pancreatic protocol contrast-enhanced computed tomography (CT) scan is performed to:
  - Confirm the presence of a mass lesion
  - Determine relationship with the superior mesenteric—portal vessels and the celiac axis
  - Evaluate for nodal disease
  - Rule out metastatic disease (liver, peritoneum, ascites, and lung).
- In the absence of a mass lesion but with dilatation of the pancreatic and common bile duct, a side-viewing endoscopy is performed to evaluate for an ampullary mass and obtain tissue for histology.
- Endoscopic ultrasound (EUS) with or without biopsy is used selectively in patients to document the presence of a lesion in case of a diagnostic dilemma, before proceeding with radical surgery.
- Preoperative biliary stenting for obstructive jaundice is performed in the setting of cholangitis, intractable pruritus, suboptimal nutritional status, liver dysfunction, and when neoadjuvant therapy is being considered.
  - Currently there is no rigid threshold of bilirubin level that mandates stenting, however, majority of patients at our center with bilirubin above 15 mg/dL are likely to undergo stenting.
- Nutritional optimization and control of comorbidities is achieved prior to surgery.
- Chest physiotherapy and nutritional supplements are included as part of a systematic prehabilitation program.

Surgical Equipment for Robotic Pancreaticoduodenectomy
- *da Vinci Xi* (Intuitive Surgical, Sunnyvale, CA, USA) Dual Console system
- Robotic ports:
    - Prograsp forceps
    - Maryland bipolar forceps
    - Curved monopolar scissors
    - Needle driver
    - Mega suture cut needle driver
    - Robotic and laparoscopic clip and hem-o-lok applicators
    - Laparoscopic Endo-GIA® staplers for bowel transections
- Energy device:
    - Harmonic Ace Scalpel (Ethicon and Johnson and Johnson) through assistant ports to reduce costs of robotic vessel-sealing device
- Preferred suture materials:
    - Synthetic, monofilament, delayed absorbable sutures:
        - Polydioxanone (PDS) 5-0 and 4-0 (Ethicon and Johnson and Johnson) with 17-mm curved needle (VISI-BLACK) depending on tissue thickness
        - The VISI- BLACK needle enables better visualization of the needle during pancreaticojejunal anastomosis, which enables correct equidistant sutures on the pancreatic duct to reduce the risk of tension and shearing forces
- Specimen extraction:
    - An indigenously prepared polyethylene extraction bag is created and used for specimen contraction, and the Alexis wound protector (Applied Medical) is used for protection of wound edges from contamination.

Patient Position for Robotic Pancreaticoduodenectomy
- The patient is positioned supine with both the arms tucked by the side of the patient.
- 30° reverse Trendelenburg position.
- An upper body convective warming blanket is used to maintain normothermia.
- The setup of equipment in the operating theater is outlined **(Fig. 1)**.

Port Position for Robotic Pancreaticoduodenectomy
- Four robotic 8-mm ports are used, each at least 8 cm apart and in a horizontal line at the level of umbilicus **(Figs. 2 and 3)**
    - *(R1)* Maryland bipolar forceps
    - *(R2)* Endoscope (Target anatomy: Uncinate process of pancreas)
    - *(R3)* Curved monopolar scissors
    - *(R4)* Prograsp forceps

Initiating Robotic Pancreaticoduodenectomy

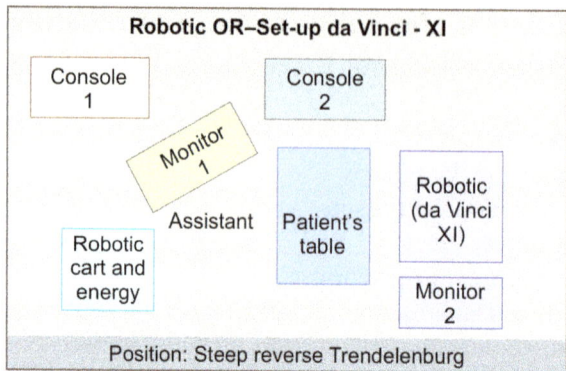

Fig. 1: OR setup for robotic pylorus preserving pancreaticoduodenectomy (PPPD).

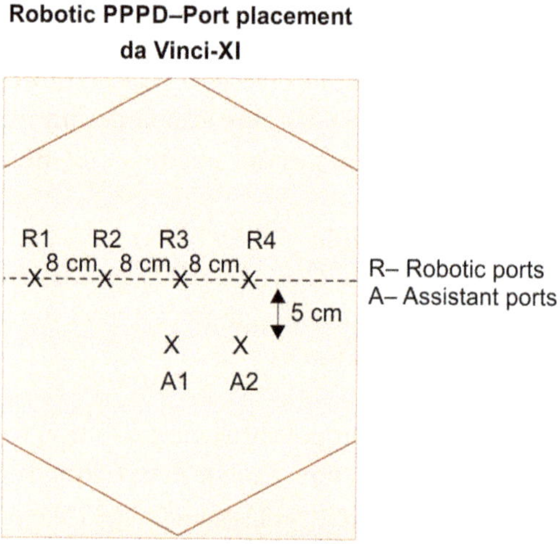

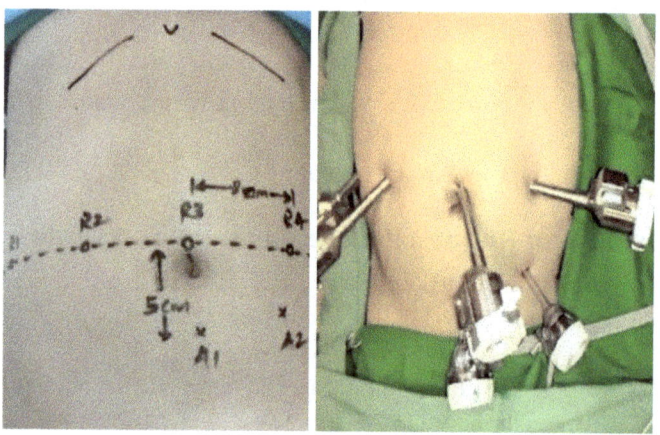

Fig. 2: Diagram showing robotic port placement for pylorus-preserving pancreaticoduodenectomy (PPPD).

Fig. 3: Robotic port placement for pylorus-preserving pancreaticoduodenectomy (PPPD).

- *(A1/A2)* Two assistant ports of 12 mm each are placed at least 5 cm below the robotic ports
  - Used for suctioning, additional retraction, clip applications, use of energy device, usage of endostaplers, delivery, and removal of gauze and needles.
- Prior to docking, staging laparoscopy can be performed to exclude presence of metastatic disease.

Operative Procedure of Robotic Pylorus-preserving Pancreaticoduodenectomy

Resection

- Exposure of the porta hepatis and opening of the gastrocolic ligament and duodenal transection
  - The falciform ligament hitch and a gallbladder fundic stitch to the anterior abdominal wall will enable optimal exposure for dissection and must be done at the start of the procedure.
  - The stomach is elevated cranially to provide tension on the gastrocolic ligament allowing division of the gastrocolic ligament and entry into the lesser sac (**Figs. 4A and B**).
  - The dissection of the gastrocolic ligament should then continue to the level of the gastric mid body, so that the omental vessels in the left half are preserved.
  - If a pylorus-preserving procedure is planned [pylorus-preserving pancreaticoduodenectomy (PPPD)], then the first part of the duodenum has to be elevated off the pancreatic head. This is done by gradually dissecting posterior to the stomach and progressing with caution until the groove between the posterior wall of the first part of duodenum and anterior surface of gastroduodenal artery (GDA) is encountered.
  - The right gastroepiploic arcade should be identified and preserved to ensure adequate vascularity of the retained pylorus at the level of the proposed transection line.
  - The right gastroepiploic vein is clipped at the confluence with the superior mesenteric vein at the inferior border of neck of the pancreas. This is done to prevent a torrential bleed from the same due to mesocolon traction as well as to facilitate uncinate dissection subsequently.
  - The middle/accessory colic veins can be traced to their insertion into the superior mesenteric vein (SMV). These may enter directly into the SMV, but commonly join the descending continuation of the right gastroepiploic vein to form the gastrocolic trunk of Henle before inserting into the SMV (**Figs. 5A and B**).

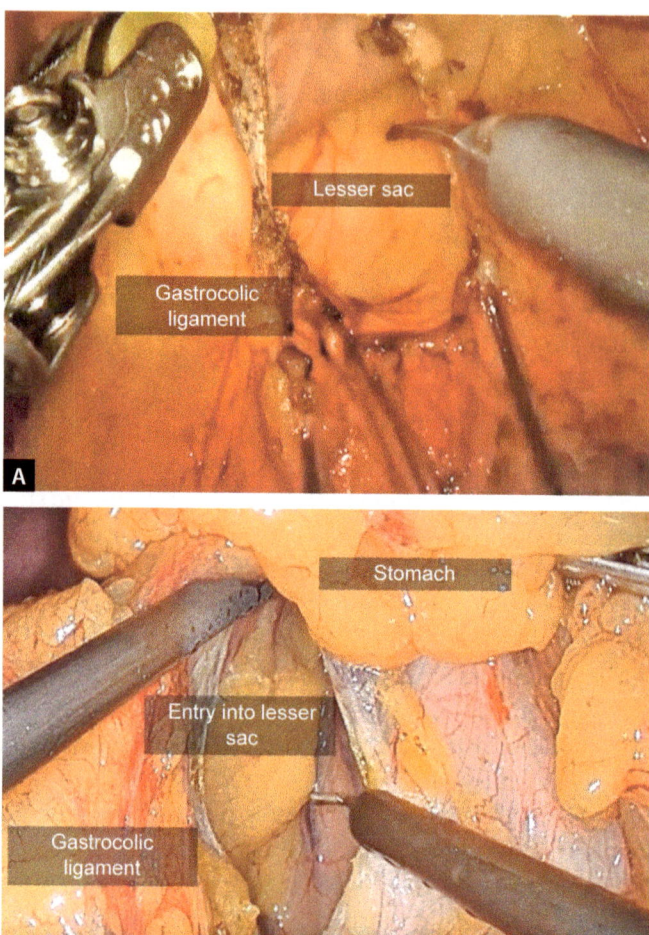

Figs. 4A and B: Robotic pancreaticoduodenectomy (RPD) versus laparoscopic pancreaticoduodenectomy (LPD)—division of gastrocolic ligament and entry into lesser sac.

- The right gastroepiploic vein is again divided at the level of the proposed duodenal transection with clips and station 6 (infrapyloric) nodes are dissected and left on the pancreatic head for retrieval with the specimen (en-bloc).
- The right gastroepiploic artery is identified by lifting the gastric antrum and careful dissection of the artery as it is given off from the GDA.
- It is usually dissected 1 cm from its origin, clipped and divided.
- The right gastric artery is identified, skeletonized, ligated, and transected at the origin with harvest of Station 5 nodes along this vessel (**Figs. 6A and B**).

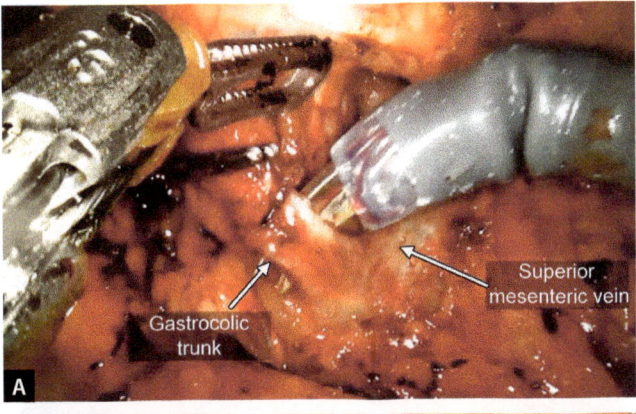
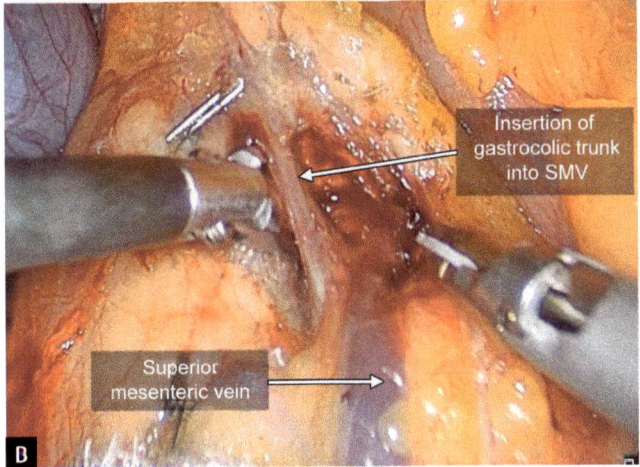

Figs. 5A and B: Robotic pancreaticoduodenectomy (RPD) versus laparoscopic pancreaticoduodenectomy (LPD)—gastrocolic trunk insertion into superior mesenteric vein (SMV).

- At this point, the duodenum is sufficiently mobilized to allow for transection using a laparoscopic linear cutting stapler with blue load.
- Transection is usually done at D1, at 1 cm distal from the pylorus when performing PPPD (**Figs. 7A to C**).
- The stomach can now be sequestered to the left of the operating field, hence allowing exposure of the suprapancreatic lymph nodes and hepatoduodenal ligament.
- Kocher maneuver:
  - The hepatic flexure is mobilized, and the right colon medially rotated to expose the SMV at the root of the small-bowel mesentery, as well as the second and third parts of the duodenum.
  - The duodenum and pancreatic head are mobilized to gain exposure of the SMA at the upper border of the left renal vein. This exposure of the SMA ensures retrieval of station 14a nodes on the right of SMA.

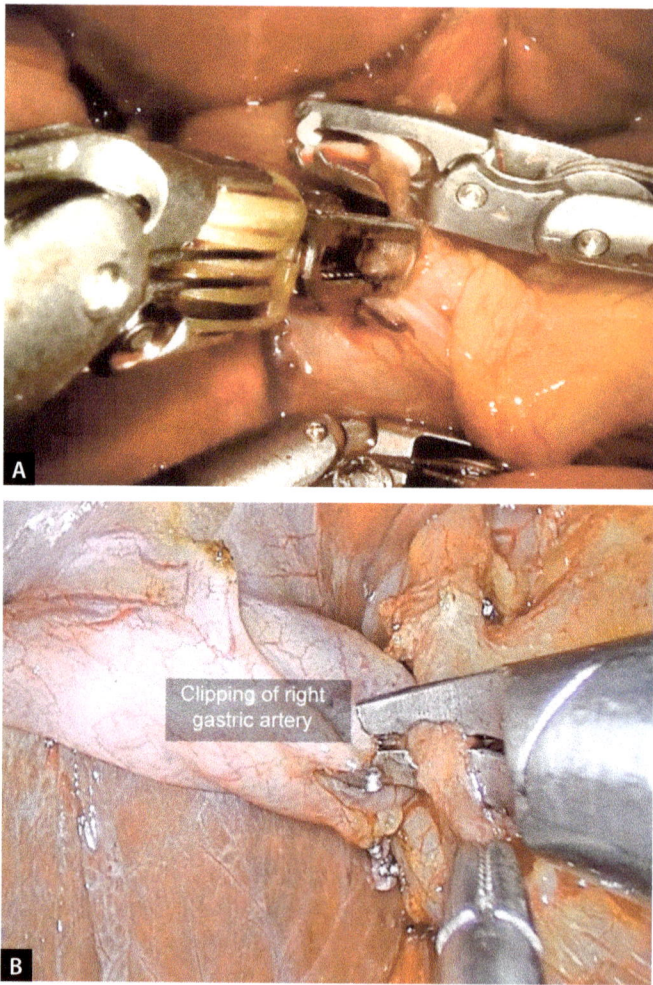

Figs. 6A and B: Robotic pancreaticoduodenectomy (RPD) versus laparoscopic pancreaticoduodenectomy (LPD): right gastric artery clipped and divided.

- Inferiorly, the Kocher maneuver is extended to mobilize the third and fourth parts of duodenum to the point that supracolic delivery of the jejunum is possible.
- The jejunum is however not divided at this juncture to avoid distension of the closed loop of bowel that can obstruct the surgical field, during uncinate process dissection later.
- Periportal dissection:
  - During hilar dissection, the vascular anatomy must be carefully assessed, in particular, the possible presence of an accessory right hepatic artery originating from the SMA.
  - The lesser omentum is incised to the left of the porta hepatis.

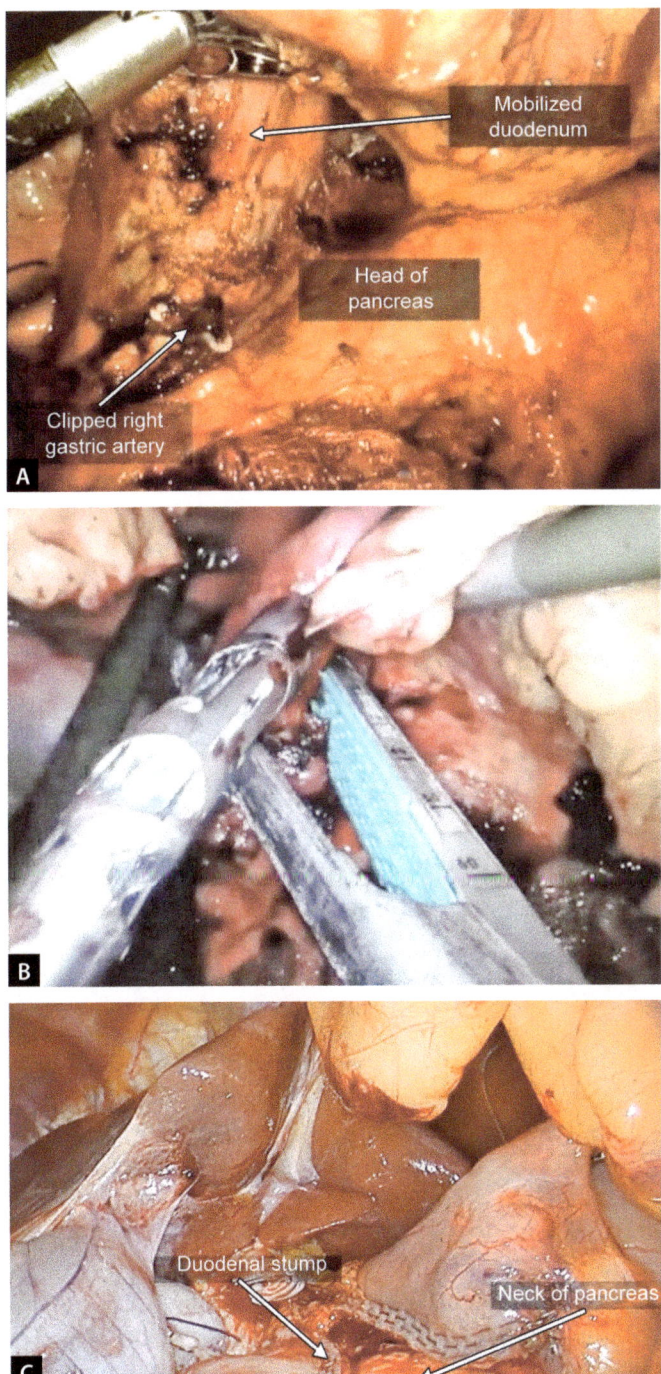

Figs. 7A to C: Mobilization and transection of duodenum.

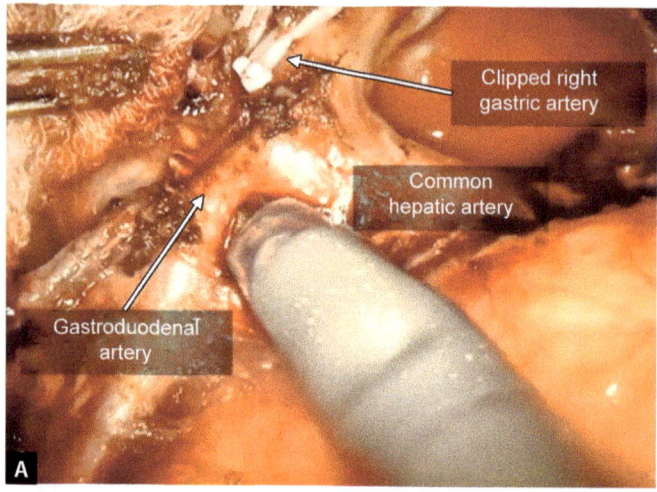
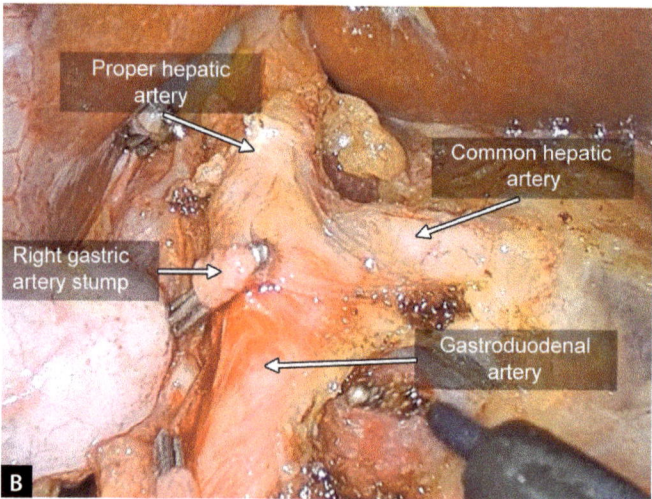

Figs. 8A and B: Robotic pancreaticoduodenectomy (RPD) versus laparoscopic pancreaticoduodenectomy (LPD)—dissection at junction of gastroduodenal artery (GDA) and common hepatic artery (CHA) at superior border of pancreas.

- Exposure of the common hepatic artery (CHA) is achieved by removal of station 8a and 8p nodes overlying the CHA above the superior border of pancreas.
- The dissection is then continued following the artery till the hepatic artery proper and the GDA (**Figs. 8A and B**).
- At this juncture, it is a useful practice to expose the portal vein just to the left of the GDA at the superior border of the pancreas neck.
- The hepatic artery is dissected superiorly till the hepatic hilum to clear the porta of station 12a and 12p nodes exposing the anterior surface and left border of portal vein (**Fig. 9**).

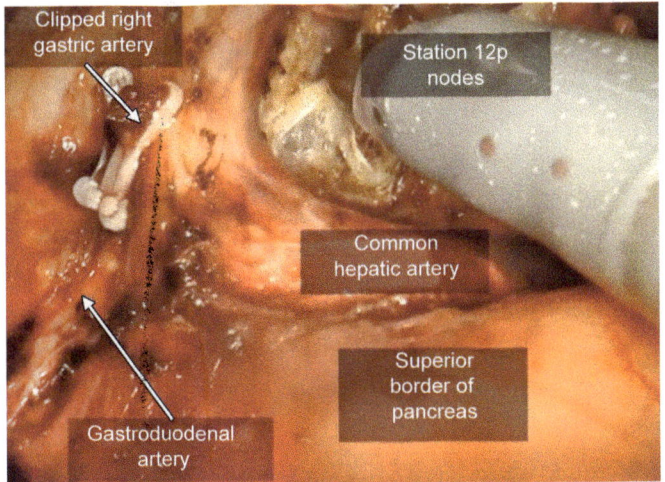

Fig. 9: Dissection of periportal nodes.

- The GDA is carefully dissected and divided between hem-o-lok clips (**Figs. 10A and B**).
- Prior to its division, it is temporarily occluded to confirm continued flow within the CHA. This can be verified by observing for visible pulsation.
- The Calot triangle is then dissected, and the cystic artery and duct are divided.
- The gallbladder mobilization is deferred in order to maintain adequate liver retraction.
- This exposes the CBD that is skeletonized by dissecting the 12b nodes to bare the right and posterior aspect of the portal vein.
- The bile duct is not divided at this juncture. This ensures that the specimen continues to hang on the bile duct, thus providing some degree of traction to the specimen during uncinate process dissection.
- Mobilization and division of pancreatic neck:
  - With exposure of the infrapancreatic SMV and suprapancreatic portal vein, a tunnel behind the neck of the pancreas, anterior to the SMV/portal vein confluence can be established with control of any small venous tributaries using clips or hemostatic device.
  - In case of inflammatory adhesions, the tunnel can be developed progressively with the transection of the pancreatic parenchyma.
  - Two hemostatic stay sutures (Prolene 4-0) are placed on both the superior and inferior margins of the pancreatic remnant.
  - Tension can be applied on the stay sutures to retract the edges of the pancreas as the transection line advances.
  - The neck of the pancreas is divided anteriorly to the portal vein using scissors and intermittent short bursts of monopolar current to

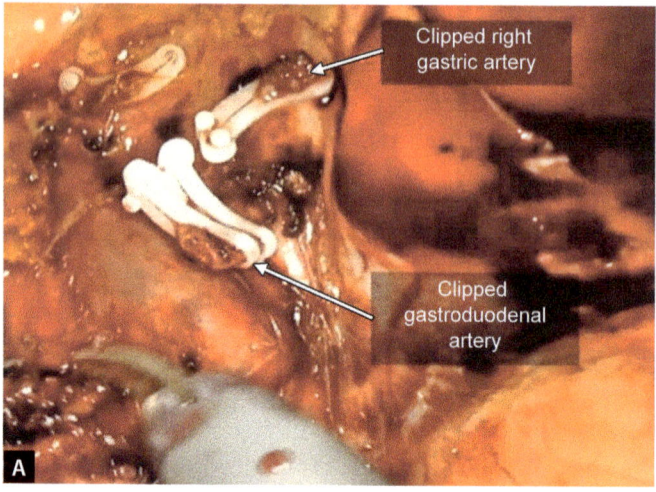

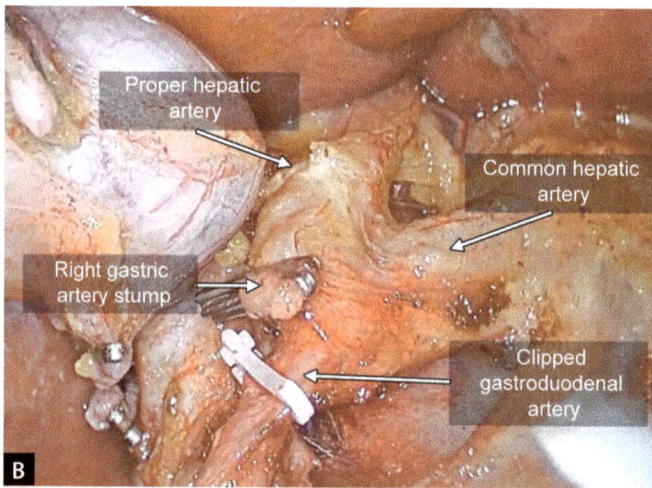

Figs. 10A and B: Robotic pancreaticoduodenectomy (RPD) versus laparoscopic pancreaticoduodenectomy (LPD)—gastroduodenal artery double-clipped and divided.

coagulate bleeding points. Mass coagulation leads to charring and can lead to lack of visibility and occlusion of a small main pancreatic duct, and should never be performed.
- Efforts should be made to identify and divide pancreatic duct under vision, 5 mm away from the pancreatic neck transection so as to facilitate placement of ductal sutures with ease during pancreaticojejunostomy (**Figs. 11A and B**).
• Uncinate dissection:
  - The approach to the uncinate process is considered the most challenging step of the resection.
  - The versatility of the robotic approach versus the laparoscopic ones are most evident during this phase which relies on the

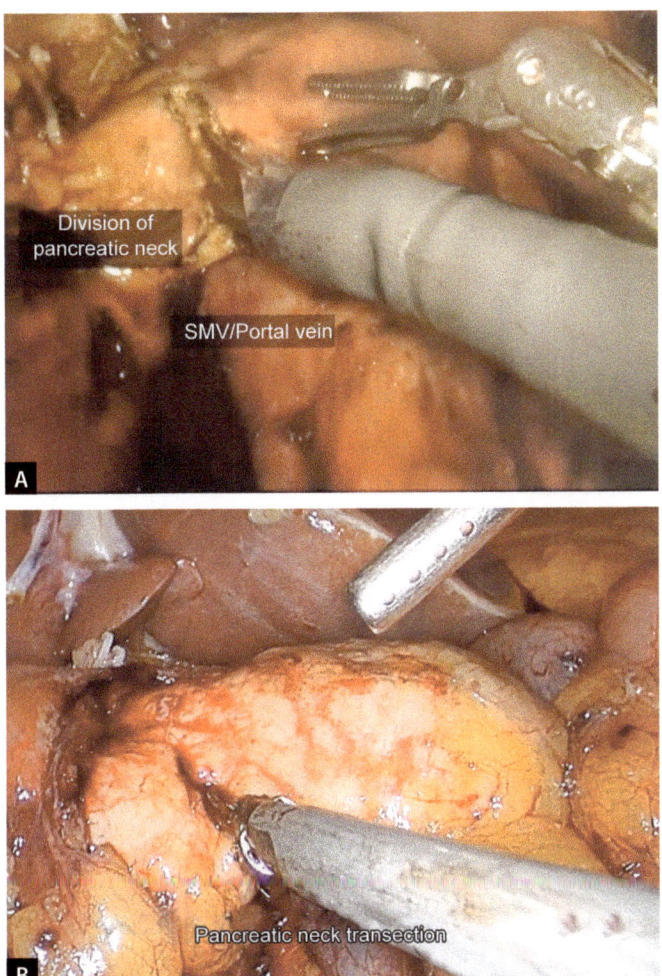

Figs. 11A and B: Robotic pancreaticoduodenectomy (RPD) versus laparoscopic pancreaticoduodenectomy (LPD)—division of pancreatic neck. (SMV: superior mesenteric vein.)

articulating movements of the robotic instruments to perform a safe dissection.
- The jejunum is divided at this point in the supracolic compartment itself.
- We prefer to use a stitch taken from lateral aspect of the duodenum and uncinate process that is brought outside the abdomen at right anterolateral region to enable varying degrees of traction that facilitates exposure during dissection of the uncinate process from the SMV initially and later from the SMA.
- With the pancreas divided, the dissection along the SMV continues proximally into the root of the small-bowel mesentery along the

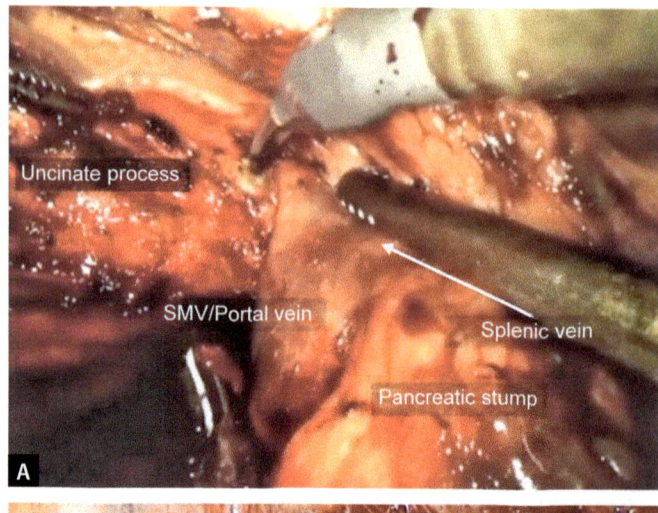

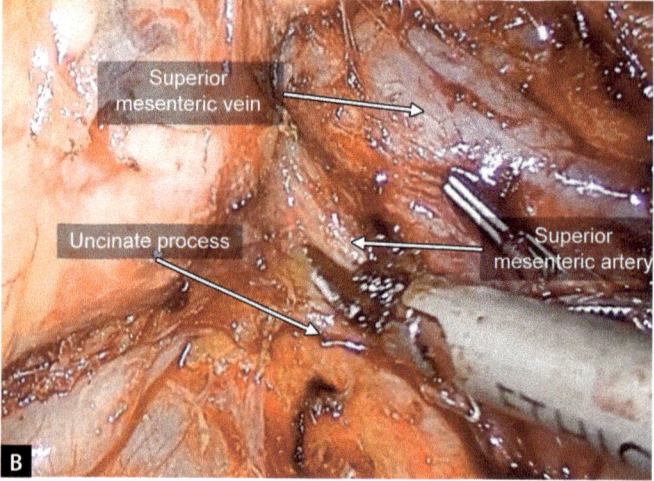

Figs. 12A and B: Robotic pancreaticoduodenectomy (RPD) uncinate dissection versus laparoscopic pancreaticoduodenectomy (LPD) uncinate dissection.
(SMV: superior mesenteric vein)

plane of Leriche to demonstrate the uncinate venous tributaries and the first jejunal vein.
- After initial dissection, the SMV is retracted with the help of ProGrasp (R4) or suction tip from the assistant port.
- Dissection along the SMV proceeds in a caudocranial direction and small branches are controlled between clips or using a sealing device.
- Venous tributaries from the first jejunal vein to the uncinate process should be treated in a similar manner.
- Exposure of the anterior surface of the SMA allows identification of the adventitia of this vessel and delineation of the mesopancreatic plane (**Figs. 12A and B**).

- As dissection progresses along the right of the SMA, lymphatics and small arteries may be encountered which are controlled with clips to prevent incidence of chyle leak.
- The origin of the inferior pancreaticoduodenal artery, once identified, is clipped, and divided.
- Ultrasonic dissector can be used on the patient side by the assistant, which can be useful during this dissection and can minimize duration of resection.
• Transection of the CBD:
  - As a last step, the bile duct is divided with cold scissors (in the case of a large fibrotic duct, diathermy may be also be used with caution).
  - Care should be taken for the right hepatic artery which may cross anterior or posterior to the bile duct or be situated to the right of the duct if replaced from the SMA.
  - The CBD division is usually performed cranial to the origin of the cystic duct which allows adequate preservation of its blood supply.
  - A bulldog clamp is placed on the proximal CBD to prevent bile contamination, while the distal end is sutured and remains attached to the specimen.
  - The specimen is placed in a plastic retrieval bag and parked in the upper abdomen.

Reconstruction

- A two-layer, end-to-side, duct-to-mucosa PJ is performed using the modified Heidelberg technique.[7]
- The jejunal limb is moved to the pancreatic cut end by a transmesocolic route or behind the root of the small bowel mesentery and prepared for the anastomosis.
- The cut surface of the pancreas is mobilized for a distance of 1–2 cm off the splenic vein to accommodate the posterior outer layer sutures.

Pancreatojejunostomy

- Posterior duct-pancreatic suture:
  - Three sutures are placed on the posterior wall of the pancreatic duct to the posterior pancreatic parenchyma.
  - The stitches are performed with 5-0 PDS 17 mm Visi-black (Ethicon®) at the 4 o'clock, 6 o'clock, and 8 o'clock positions.
  - The suture starts into the pancreatic duct traversing the full thickness of the parenchyma, until the posterior wall of the pancreas (from inside to outside) **(Fig. 13)**.
- Anterior duct-pancreatic suture:
  - Three identical full-thickness sutures are passed from the anterior pancreatic parenchyma to the anterior wall of the pancreatic duct in

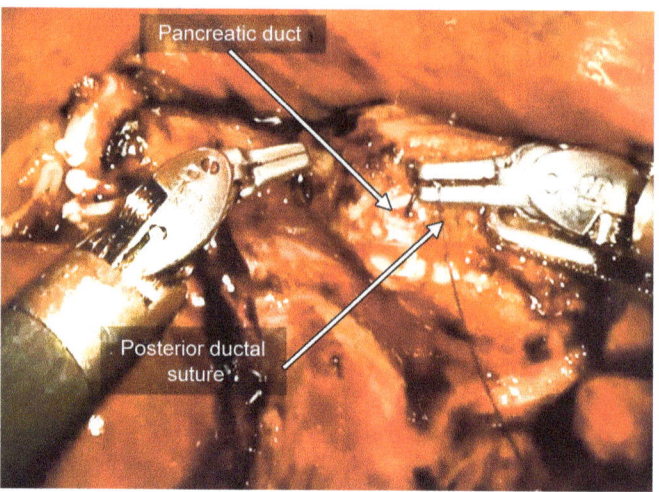

Fig. 13: Posterior duct suture @ 6 o'clock.

  a similar fashion at the 10 o'clock, 12 o'clock, and 2 o'clock positions (from outside to inside).
  - The posterior and anterior duct-pancreatic sutures remain untied and may be temporarily clipped and retracted to the left of the surgical field.
- Posterior outer layer:
  - The antimesenteric border of the jejunum is oriented to lie along the posterior aspect of the pancreatic stump.
  - The seromuscular layer of the jejunal wall is sutured to the posterior surface of the pancreatic capsule using interrupted 5-0 PDS suture (**Figs. 14A and B**).
  - Usually up to 4–5 sutures are required for the posterior outer layer.
- Posterior inner layer:
  - A 5-mm enterotomy is made at the antimesenteric surface of the jejunum using electrocautery at a position that allows easy apposition with the exposed pancreatic duct.
  - The posterior duct sutures can now be retrieved and sutured with full thickness of the jejunum along the inferior edge of the enterotomy at corresponding positions, then securely knotted (**Figs. 15A and B**).
- Stenting of pancreatic duct:
  - If a stent is deemed necessary, it can be placed at this time.
  - A plastic stent, 20 cm long, is inserted into the pancreatic duct and allowed to extend up to 15 cm into the jejunal lumen (**Figs. 16A and B**).

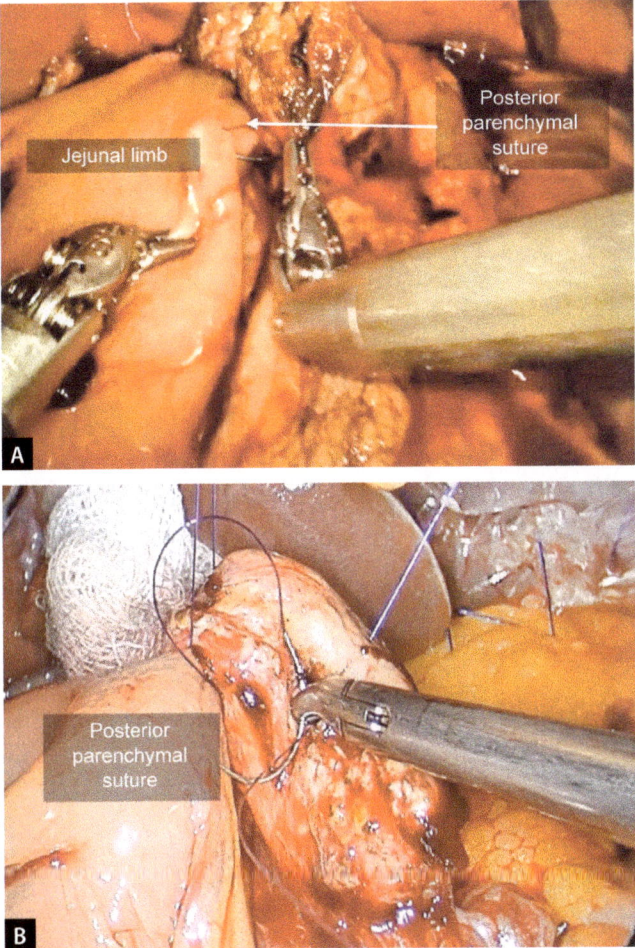

Figs. 14A and B: Robotic pancreaticoduodenectomy (RPD) versus laparoscopic pancreaticoduodenectomy (LPD)—posterior outer layer suture.

- Anterior inner layer:
    - The anterior duct sutures in the 10 o'clock, 12 o'clock, and 2 o'clock positions are now passed in similar full thickness fashion to the superior edge of the enterotomy and knotted (**Fig. 17**).
- Anterior outer layer:
    - An interrupted suture is performed using 5-0 PDS suture, anchoring the seromuscular layer of the jejunum to the anterior aspect of the pancreatic capsule, similar to that performed at the posterior outer layer (**Figs. 18A and B**).
- Jejunal stay suture:
    - The two previously placed hemostatic sutures on the superior and inferior edges of the remnant pancreatic stump are passed to the jejunal seromuscular layer and tied.

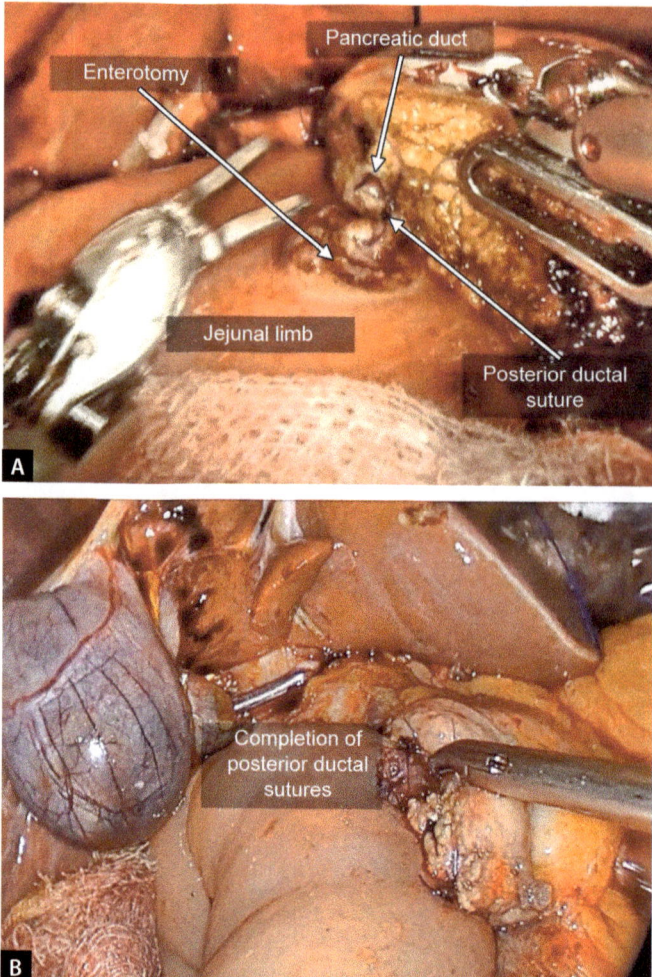

Figs. 15A and B: Robotic pancreaticoduodenectomy (RPD) versus laparoscopic pancreaticoduodenectomy (LPD) posterior duct layer.

Hepaticojejunostomy

- The hepaticojejunostomy (HJ) is carried out in an end-to-side fashion (**Figs. 19A and B**).
- A redundant loop of jejunum is maintained between the PJ and HJ anastomosis to ensure no tension ensuring at least 15 cm between the biliary and pancreatic anastomosis.
- Interrupted 4/0 or 5/0 PDS sutures are placed along the anterior and posterior layers of the cut end of the bile duct at 1 mm intervals and secured with clips without being tied to prevent displacement.
- An enterotomy is made close to the mesenteric border of the jejunal loop, which is no larger than 50% the diameter of the duct.

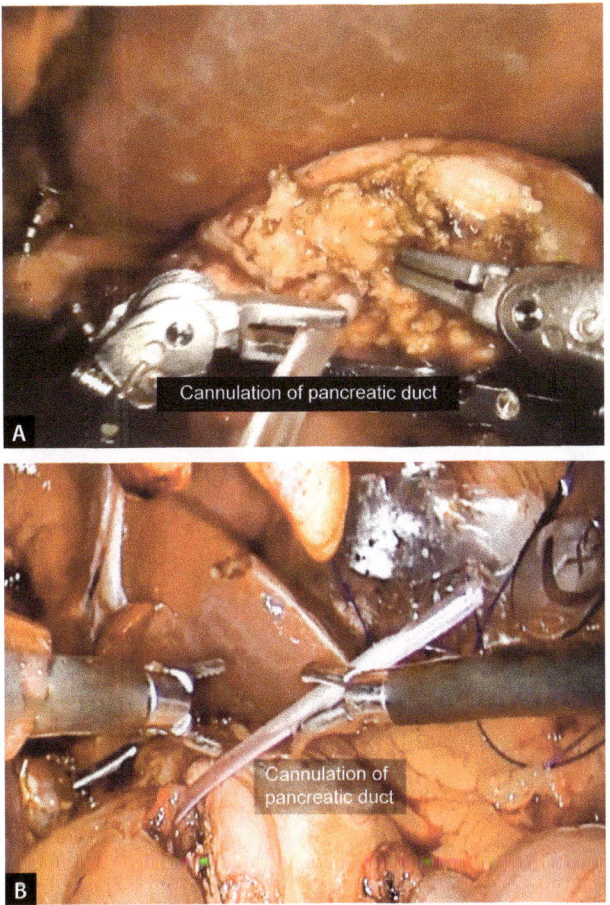

Figs. 16A and B: Robotic pancreaticoduodenectomy (RPD) versus laparoscopic pancreaticoduodenectomy (LPD)—cannulation of pancreatic duct.

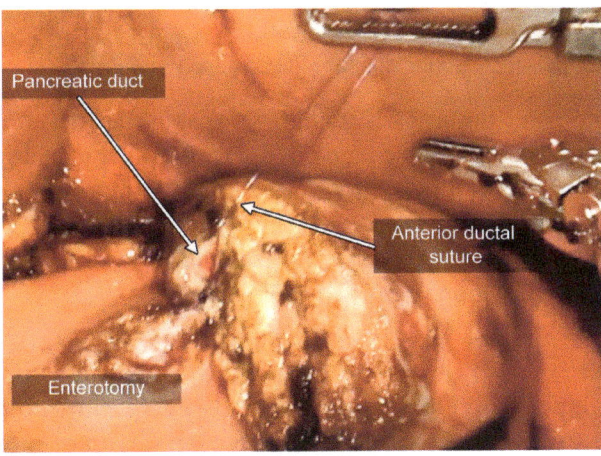

Fig. 17: Anterior duct layer.

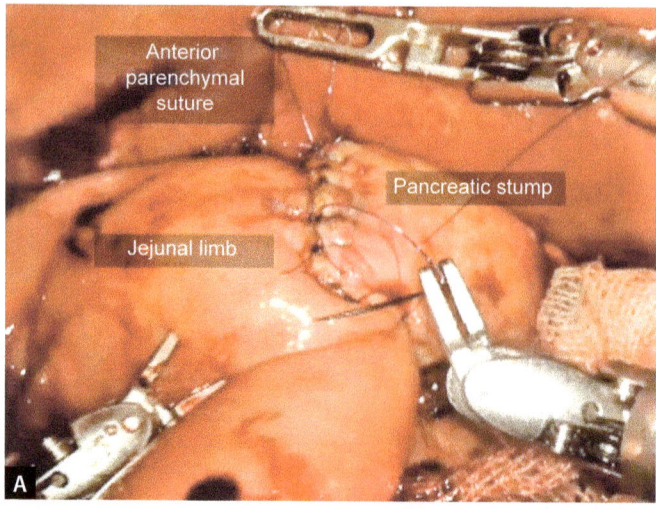

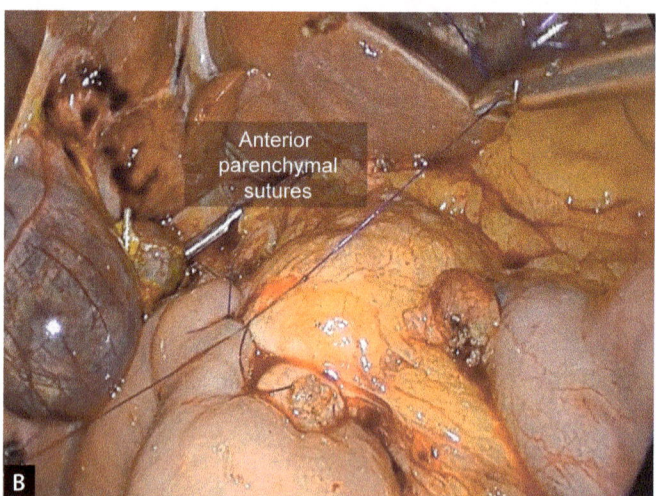

Figs. 18A and B: Robotic pancreaticoduodenectomy (RPD) versus laparoscopic pancreaticoduodenectomy (LPD)—anterior outer layer.

- The anterior and posterior duct sutures are passed into the corresponding ends of the enterotomy and knotted to ensure a water tight anastomosis.
- Alternatively, a running suture can be used for this anastomosis if the duct is wide enough.
- A surgical gauze can be placed at the posterior surface of the anastomosis and inspected later on to ensure no bile staining.

Pylorus/Gastrojejunostomy

- A 6–7 cm upper midline incision is made for specimen retrieval and through the same, an end-to-side antecolic duodenojejunostomy is performed.

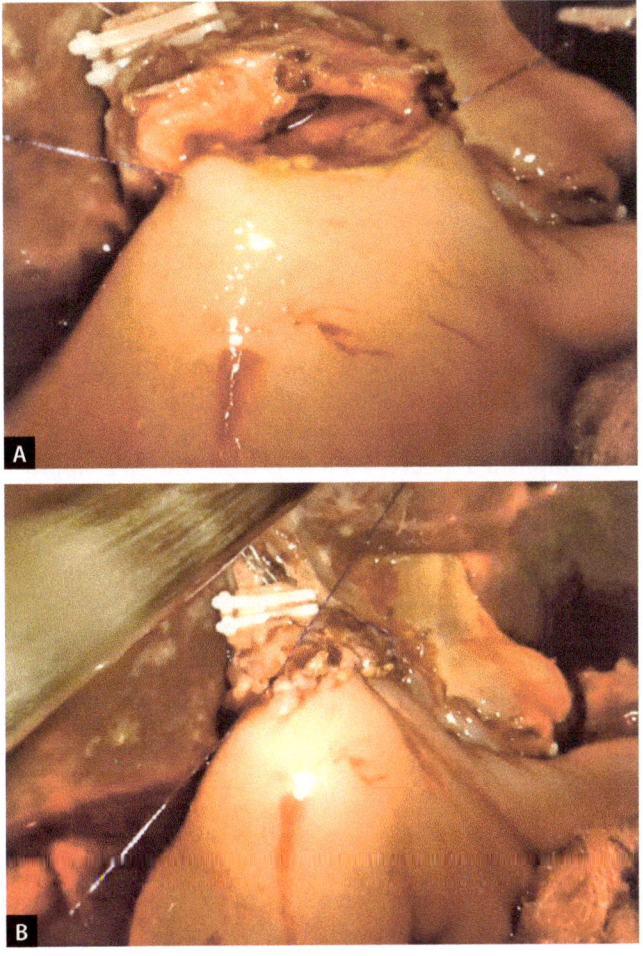

Figs. 19A and B: Hepaticojejunostomy.

- This is fashioned along the same loop of jejunum, in two layers with 4-0 continuous PDS sutures at least 40 cm distal to the bilioenteric anastomosis.
- If needed, a nasojejunal tube is placed across the duodenal anastomosis for postoperative enteral feeding, should delayed gastric emptying ensue.

Extraction of the Specimen and Closure

- The specimen is extracted through the abdominal incision.
- Alternative extraction sites may be considered in case of previous abdominal surgery.
- *Two flat drains are placed:* One right drain posterior to the biliary anastomosis and a left drain anterior to the pancreatic anastomosis.
- The drains are cut to a length such that a shortest route is used for egressing of drained fluids.

Key Differences between Robotic and Laparoscopic Pancreaticoduodenectomy in Operative Technique

- The standard benefits of robotic platform over the laparoscopic approach include better ergonomics, improved dexterity and range of motion, tremor filtration, and a shorter learning curve.
- The disadvantages of robotic approach include high initial cost, maintenance cost, and higher surgery expenditure for the patients.
- Long docking time is a potential disadvantage with robotic surgery.
- Both techniques have shown to reduce postoperative pain, have earlier functional recovery, and decrease hospital stay.
- Perioperative wound infections and the risk of incisional hernia are significantly lower compared to the open approach.
- In terms of operative technique, portal lymphadenectomy is easier and can be accomplished quicker with RPD than with LPD approach, due to greater range of motion and maneuverability.
- The uncinate dissection is extremely important to achieve a negative margin especially in pancreatic head carcinoma or ampullary carcinoma with a significant pancreatic invasion. Due to the endowrist action, it is easier to reach the SMA underneath the SMV during uncinate first and SMA first techniques, which may result in superior oncological outcomes. This may also enable superior clearance of the mesopancreas.
- Superior magnification, control of the camera, and greater dexterity of the operating surgeon can be instrumental in clipping small vessels from the SMV and SMA.
- The surgeon will be more efficient at the uncinate dissection by remaining just to the right side of the SMA, thereby preventing pancreatic parenchyma transection and decreasing blood loss in the process.
- Pancreaticojejunal anastomotic techniques can be a major source of perioperative morbidity and mortality. Due to the finesse of the robotic instruments, the posterior inner and anterior inner ductal sutures can be placed with greater accuracy avoiding inadvertent narrowing of the main pancreatic duct.
- The versatility of the robotic arms ensures that when pancreatic sutures are taken, the needle does not cause microscopic shearing forces and prevents "cut through" which may translate into lesser clinically relevant pancreatic fistulas. This is more frequent when dealing with a soft pancreas.
- In the RPD approach, superior ergonomics and lesser surgeon fatigue can prevent inadvertent rough handling of the pancreatic stump during the pancreaticoenteric anastomosis.
- Standardization of open surgical techniques can be replicated on the robotic platform with much more precision, than with the laparoscopic approach.
- Hence, the robotic approach negates the deficiencies of the laparoscopic technique and can result in similar perioperative results, oncological clearance, and survival whilst enabling earlier functional recovery.

EVIDENCE FOR MINIMALLY INVASIVE PANCREATICODUOENECTOMY

- Adequate and extensive experience in open PD is a prerequisite before attempting MIPD.
- The robot provides enhanced skills to surgeons, hence results in a superior experience, especially for finer and more meticulous dissection and suturing.
- Ergonomic benefits afforded to the surgeon will likely decrease fatigue in the operating room and could translate into improved outcomes.
- Presently, the main factors against widespread adoption of robotic PD are:
  - High costs involved
  - The ability of surgeons to navigate the learning curve that is perhaps possible only in dedicated centers of experience
  - Lack of evidence clearly supporting equivalence/superiority of robotic over open PD.
- Safety outcomes for the individual patient must not be compromised upon, during the learning curve phase of the robotic PD.

EVIDENCE FOR ROBOTIC PANCREATICODUODENECTOMY VERSUS OPEN PANCREATICODUODENECTOMY

- Randomized control trials comparing RPD to open pancreaticoduodenectomy (OPD) are lacking, and major evidence is based on retrospective series data. Hence, due to the possibility of confounding variables and inherent selection bias, the strength of recommendation for RPD is limited.
- In 2013, comprising 132 robotic PDs, Zeh and Moser showed safety and feasibility of RPD compared to LPD and OPD. There was a low incidence of conversion. They did not find any significant difference in the length of stay, but operative times were significantly higher.[8]
- Chalikonda et al. demonstrated that patients who underwent robotic PD had a significantly shorter length of stay when compared to open PD.[9]
- Most studies show similar morbidity and complications but one study showed significantly lower complication rate following robotic PD (25 vs. 75%, $p = 0.05$).[10]
- Most studies show similar lymph node retrieval with the robotic approach when compared to open,[9,10] but one series showed statistically significant improvement in lymph node yield.[11]
- Analysis of retrospective studies of RPD versus OPD showed conversion rates ranging from 2 to 16%. Operative time was significantly longer in all but one study with mean operative times for RPD ranging from 410 to 549 minutes. Estimated blood loss was significantly less for RPD in all but one study.[12-16]

FORMAL TRAINING IN MINIMALLY INVASIVE PANCREATICODUODENECTOMY

- It is imperative for surgeons to have adequate experience in OPD before embarking upon MIPD.
- Enrolment into structured training program is strongly recommended which includes virtual reality simulation, biotissue models to practice dissection, anastomotic techniques, and surgical video review.
- On-site proctoring by experienced minimal invasive pancreatic surgeon, during the learning curve can ensure patient safety and have comparable outcomes to the standard OPD.
- In LPD learning curve, related improvements in outcome were seen after 10–50 cases.[17-20]
- For RPD, 20–40 cases have been described as needed to overcome the learning curve.[21-23]
- A few high-volume experienced centers have reported excellent outcomes, whilst some have reported suboptimal and some have reported poor outcomes with the minimal invasive approach.
- Hence, optimal case selection, a stepwise and staggered approach initially with a lower threshold to convert to open in case of failure to progress, is best suited to those teams which are planning to get into MIPD.

CONCLUSION

- There is insufficient data at present to routinely recommend MIPD over OPD. Centers performing MIPD should include all of their MIPD outcomes data into national and international registries, and prospectively maintained databases. To facilitate comparative analysis, additional randomized trials comparing LPD and RPD to OPD are encouraged. Trials should be performed only in centers where the MIPD learning curve has been completed.
- When MIPD is performed, evidence suggests that the incidence of pancreatic leak is equivalent to the open approach, but this may vary depending on case selection. A higher leak rate can be anticipated when employed for ampullary and duodenal tumors, which tend to be associated with nondilated pancreatic duct and soft pancreatic texture. Hence, fistula rate may be falsely elevated in this group of patients undergoing LPD/RPD when compared to historical controls of open PD surgery.
- Most studies indicate less blood loss and better functional results (pain, earlier recovery, discharge from hospital), but longer operative times.
- Similar complication rate, morbidity, and mortality are documented.
- Rates of R0 resection, nodal retrieval, and time to adjuvant therapy initiation are shown to be equivalent, although long-term survival studies are still pending.

- Wound complications and chance of incisional hernia subsequently will be less with minimally invasive approaches.
- Length of hospital stay usually depends on surgical complications such as hemorrhage, bile leak, pancreatic fistula, delayed gastric emptying, and chyle leak. Hence, the apparent tendency for early discharge of patients who undergo MIPD cannot be attributed to a lower incidence of complications, which is documented to be similar between the two groups. Therefore, it can be postulated that only a small subset of patients who have no specific surgical complications and stay longer due to pain-related or wound-related complications seem to benefit from MIPD compared to OPD approaches.
- Further refinement in robotic and laparoscopic technology and instrumentation, standardization of surgical techniques, centralization of MIPD to high-volume centers may result in defining its role in the future. At this stage, MIPD especially LPD remains investigational.
- Robotic PD appears promising given its advantages, especially for reconstruction, and it will continue to be evaluated further in the coming years.

REFERENCES

1. Traverso LW, Longmire WP. Preservation of the pylorus in pancreaticoduodenectomy. Surg Gynecol Obstet. 1978;146(6):959-62.
2. Shrikhande SV, Sivasanker M, Vollmer CM, Friess H, Besselink MG, Fingerhut A, et al. Pancreatic anastomosis after pancreatoduodenectomy: a position statement by the International Study Group of Pancreatic Surgery (ISGPS). 2017;161(9):1221-34.
3. Crist DW, Sitzmann JV, Cameron JL. Improved hospital morbidity, mortality, and survival after the Whipple procedure. Ann Surg. 1987;206(3):358-65.
4. Shrikhande SV, Shinde RS, Chaudhari VA, Kurunkar SR, Desouza AL, Agarwal V, et al. Twelve hundred consecutive pancreato-duodenectomies from single centre: impact of centre of excellence on pancreatic cancer surgery across India. World J Surg. 2019;44(8):2784-93.
5. Gagner M, Pomp A. Laparoscopic pylorus-preserving pancreatoduodenectomy. Surg Endosc. 1994;8(5):408-10.
6. Giulianotti PC, Coratti A, Angelini M, Sbrana F, Cecconi S, Balestracci T, et al. Robotics in general surgery: personal experience in a large community hospital. Arch Surg. 2003;138(7):777-84.
7. Shrikhande SV, Kleeff J, Büchler MW, Friess H. Pancreatic anastomosis after pancreaticoduodenectomy: how we do it. Indian Journal of Surgery, Volume 69. New Delhi: Springer; 2007. pp. 224-9.
8. Zureikat AH, Moser AJ, Boone BA, Bartlett DL, Zenati M, Zeh HJ. 250 robotic pancreatic resections safety and feasibility. Ann Surg. 2013;258(4):554-9; discussion 559-62.
9. Chalikonda S, Aguilar-Saavedra JR, Walsh RM. Laparoscopic robotic-assisted pancreaticoduodenectomy: a case-matched comparison with open resection. Surg Endosc [Internet]. 2012;26(9):2397–402.

10. Zhou N, Chen J, Liu Q, Zhang X, Wang Z, Ren S, et al. Outcomes of pancreatoduodenectomy with robotic surgery versus open surgery. Int J Med Robot Comput Assist Surg. 2011;7(2):131-7.
11. Buchs NC, Addeo P, Bianco FM, Ayloo S, Benedetti E, Giulianotti PC. Robotic versus open pancreaticoduodenectomy: a comparative study at a single institution. World J Surg [Internet]. 2011;35(12):2739-46.
12. Baker EH, Ross SW, Seshadri R, Swan RZ, Iannitti DA, Vrochides D, et al. Robotic pancreaticoduodenectomy for pancreatic adenocarcinoma: role in 2014 and beyond. Journal of Gastrointestinal Oncology, Volume 6. Pioneer Bioscience Publishing; 2015. pp. 396-405.
13. Bao PQ, Mazirka PO, Watkins KT. Retrospective comparison of robot-assisted minimally invasive versus open pancreaticoduodenectomy for periampullary neoplasms. J Gastrointest Surg. 2014;18(4):682-9.
14. Chen S, Chen JZ, Zhan Q, Deng XX, Shen BY, Peng CH, et al. Robot-assisted laparoscopic versus open pancreaticoduodenectomy: a prospective, matched, mid-term follow-up study. Surg Endosc. 2015;29(12):3698-711.
15. Lai ECH, Yang GPC, Tang CN. Robot-assisted laparoscopic pancreaticoduodenectomy versus open pancreaticoduodenectomy - a comparative study. Int J Surg. 2012;10(9):475-9.
16. Kim SC, Song KB, Jung YS, Kim YH, Park DH, Lee SS, et al. Short-term clinical outcomes for 100 consecutive cases of laparoscopic pylorus-preserving pancreatoduodenectomy: improvement with surgical experience. Surg Endosc. 2013;27(1):95-103.
17. Nagakawa Y, Nakamura Y, Honda G, Gotoh Y, Ohtsuka T, Ban D, et al. Learning curve and surgical factors influencing the surgical outcomes during the initial experience with laparoscopic pancreaticoduodenectomy. J Hepatobiliary Pancreat Sci. 2018;25(11):498-507.
18. Speicher PJ, Nussbaum DP, White RR, Zani S, Mosca PJ, Blazer DG, et al. Defining the learning curve for team-based laparoscopic pancreaticoduodenectomy. Ann Surg Oncol. 2014;21(12):4014-9.
19. Wang M, Meng L, Cai Y, Li Y, Wang X, Zhang Z, et al. Learning curve for laparoscopic pancreaticoduodenectomy: a CUSUM analysis. J Gastrointest Surg. 2016;20(5):924-35.
20. Shyr BU, Chen SC, Shyr YM, Wang SE. Learning curves for robotic pancreatic surgery-from distal pancreatectomy to pancreaticoduodenectomy. Med (United States). 2018;97(45).
21. Takahashi C, Shridhar R, Huston J, Meredith K. Outcomes associated with robotic approach to pancreatic resections. J Gastrointest Oncol. 2018;9(5):936-41.
22. Boone BA, Zenati M, Hogg ME, Steve J, Moser AJ, Bartlett DL, et al. Assessment of quality outcomes for robotic pancreaticoduodenectomy: identification of the learning curve. JAMA Surg. 2015;150(5):416-22.
23. Asbun HJ, Moekotte AL, Vissers FL, Kunzler F, Cipriani F, Alseidi A, et al. The Miami International Evidence-based Guidelines on minimally invasive pancreas resection. Ann Surg. 2020;271(1):1-14.

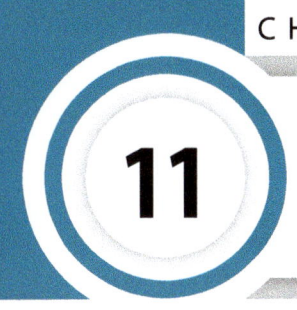

CHAPTER 11

Minimally Invasive Distal Pancreatectomy

Christoph Berchtold, Thilo Hackert

INTRODUCTION

While pioneers of minimally invasive surgery early attempted all types of pancreatic resection, the adaptation of laparoscopic techniques was slower than in other fields of abdominal surgery. Subsequently mainly enucleation and distal pancreatectomy gained wider acceptance because these procedures are technically easier compared to pancreatoduodenectomy and there is no need to create anastomoses.[1,2] Despite lack of high-quality studies and low level of evidence, the published opinion has been in favor of a minimally invasive approach to distal pancreatectomy for quite a while.[2] A recent analysis of hospital data from USA shows that almost two-thirds of distal pancreatectomies were performed minimally invasively, yet with a large interhospital variation from 0 to 100% of suitable cases.[3]

As with other minimally invasive procedures, minimally invasive distal pancreatectomy (MIDP) has not been introduced into clinical practice as a consequence of controlled trials assessing risk and benefit. Yet, large scale observations have shown a trend to better perioperative outcomes with reduced blood loss and shorter length of hospital stay.[4-6] Taking into consideration that evidence is of low quality, authors concluded that MIDP seemed to be safe and effective compared to open surgery, but the question of oncological efficacy and long-term equivalence remained open.[4-6] Meanwhile two randomized controlled trials have verified the advantages of MIDP for short-term postoperative outcomes.[7-9] Likewise, data about reduced major morbidity accumulated indicating a risk reduction following implementation of MIDP instead of open distal pancreatectomy (ODP).[10]

Observational studies have found that factors disposing surgeons to favor MIDP were benign tumors, smaller tumor size, higher body mass index (BMI), whereas patients with ODP had higher American Society of Anesthesiologists (ASA) classification, malign tumors, and needed more often extended (multivisceral) resection.[3,11] As successful operations have been reported for many situations considered initially as contraindication for a minimally invasive approach such as vascular resection or prior upper abdominal surgery, the selection mainly depends on the individual surgeon's experience and preferences.[12-14] Accordingly, there is no consensus about criteria to exclude patients from an attempt at MIDP.[15]

In the last years, research has focused on oncologic outcomes. A large multi-institutional retrospective cohort study in Europe (DIPLOMA) confirmed short-term clinical advantages of MIDP versus ODP.[16] While overall survival was comparable between the two approaches, results of specific oncological endpoints were different in opposite ways with higher R0-resection rate but lower lymph node retrieval and resection of Gerota fascia in MIDP.[16,17] A systematic review and meta-analysis of existing studies found comparable results for survival and R0-resection rate but could not resolve the problem of a possible treatment allocation bias which would preclude a firm conclusion about oncologic equivalence.[18] For pancreatic neuroendocrine tumors, comparable oncologic outcomes including long-term survival have been published.[19]

It is difficult to estimate how many distal pancreatectomies are performed by a minimally invasive approach. Results from a large registry in USA have recently shown that a majority (64.5%) of (partly selected) cases were done as MIDP with a quarter using robotic technique.[3] Yet, the variation between hospital-level use was remarkably high (median 69%, range 0–100%). Nevertheless, it seems easy to predict that the numbers of MIDP will increase steadily as well as the proportion of robotic compared to laparoscopic procedures.[2]

STANDARD OPERATIVE TECHNIQUE FOR LAPAROSCOPIC DISTAL PANCREATOSPLENECTOMY

While the principal operative steps in distal pancreatectomy are similar in minimally invasive and open surgery technical considerations seem to play a bigger role in using a minimally invasive approach to overcome the inherent shortcomings of laparoscopy and make the procedure as safe as possible.

We prefer the so-called "French position" and—like most authors—use as standard four trocars placed in a transverse curved line in the upper abdomen with an additional fifth trocar in the epigastrium.[20] The operation starts with a wide dissection of the gastrocolic ligament giving way into the lesser sac and mobilization of the left colon flexure. The gastrocolic ligament is divided just below the gastroepiploic vessels and the greater omentum is not detached from the transverse colon to avoid the need for retraction of a bulky omentum into a cranial direction. We use a vessel sealing device either with bipolar coagulation or ultrasound. The stomach is retracted ventrally and to the right either by a retractor or two percutaneous sutures through the dorsal gastric wall. After visualization of the pancreas and the tumor, the extent of the necessary resection can be assessed. When a splenectomy is to be done, the short gastric vessels are dissected as far as the left crus of diaphragm. The superior mesenteric vein is exposed at the lower margin of the pancreatic body. By meticulous dissection, the vein is separated from the

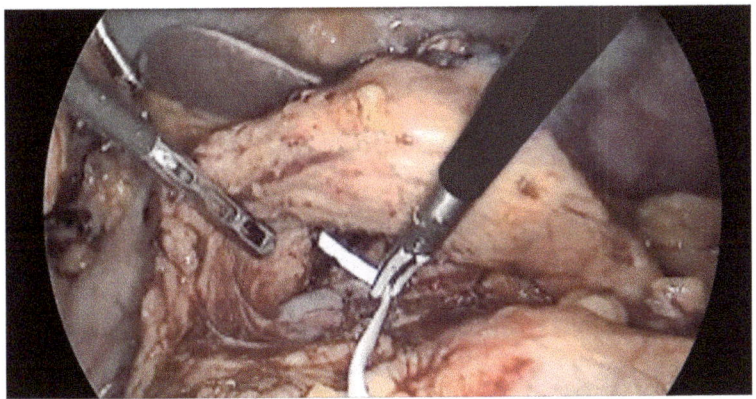

Fig. 1: Preparation of dorsal side of pancreas and splenic vein.

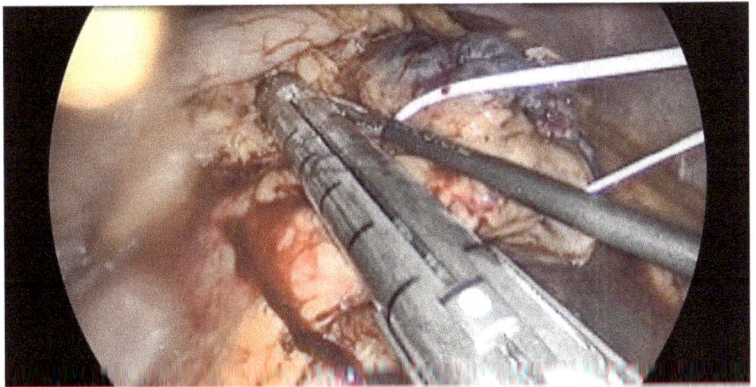

Fig. 2: Stapler division of pancreas.

backside of the pancreas until the instrument crosses behind the pancreas and the tunnel of the planned transection line is completed. It is important to pay attention to the splenic artery at the upper margin of the pancreas. Vessel loops are placed both around the pancreas and the splenic artery **(Fig 1)**. After enlarging the retropancreatic space, the pancreas can be divided by an endoscopic stapling device. Mostly we use a 60 mm "thick" cartridge, in case of a thin and soft pancreas a "medium" cartridge **(Fig 2)**. We do not use any type of staple line enforcement. The splenic artery must be clearly identified to avoid the mistake of confounding and inadvertently dividing the hepatic artery. Sometimes both the vein and the artery can be cut using one vascular stapling device.

Otherwise, we would prefer to divide the artery first by at least two clips proximally and one distally **(Fig 3)**. Same can be done with the vein, but we would prefer to cut it with a vascular stapler. If the splenic vessels cannot be safely separated, en-bloc stapling together with the pancreas can be done

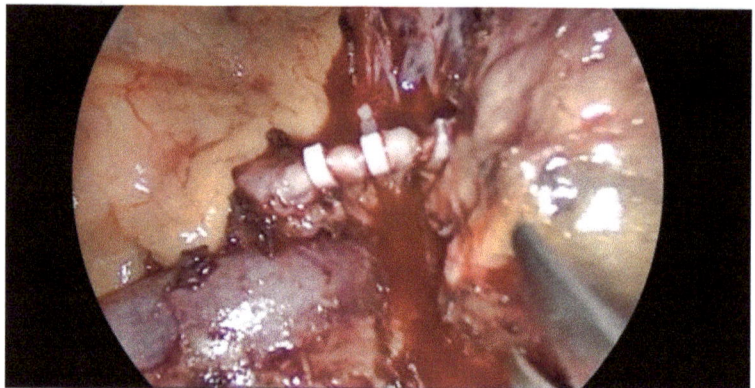

Fig. 3: Division of the splenic artery.

when the dissection plane is in safe distance left off the venous confluence and celiac axis. The dissection continues in a mediolateral direction. Depending on the size and extent of the tumor, the dissection plane can be chosen according to the RAMPS concept. If an adrenalectomy is necessary, the suprarenal vein must be exposed and divided, and care must be taken not to harm the renal vessels. In the retroperitoneal space, we can usually progress in a vessel-free plane until the splenic hilum is reached from behind. The attachments of the spleen to the diaphragm are divided by smoothly lifting up the spleen from the lower pole upward. The specimen is placed in a large bag. If indicated, we perform a cholecystectomy. While we regularly cover the pancreatic stump with a ligamentum teres—patch in open surgery, we mostly go without because we do not feel comfortable stitching the pancreas with laparoscopic instruments. The extraction is usually made through a 5-6 cm transverse minilaparotomy above the symphysis. After closure of the incision, the pneumoperitoneum is reestablished, the situs flushed with warm saline and checked for hemostasis. We do not principally drain the abdomen but leave this to the discretion of the surgeon. After extraction of the trocars under view and desufflation, the incisions are closed.

The technique described is similar to that published recently by a group of international experts.[21] The standardized procedure with a determined sequence of procedural steps seems to attribute to good outcomes. We would also emphasize the usefulness of a "progressive stepwise compression technique" of stapling but question the benefit of "staple line reinforcement."[4]

■ SPECIAL SURGICAL CONSIDERATIONS

It is not proven yet that a more radical approach to distal pancreatectomy like "radical antegrade modular pancreatosplenectomy (RAMPS)" produces superior oncologic results compared to the conventional approach.[22] Nevertheless, the technical feasibility and oncological safety of minimally invasive RAMPS have been shown in selected cases and criteria for proper selection considering extent and location of the tumor have been proposed ("Yonsei criteria").[23]

While most surgeons would agree that locally advanced tumors with the potential need of multivisceral resections still are a domain of open surgery, there have been reports of minimally invasive extended resections.[12,13,24] Conversion rate expectedly seems to be higher, whereas morbidity and mortality were comparable with "standard" MIDP.[24] A final judgement or general recommendation is not possible because of small numbers reported and selection bias regarding treatment allocation.

For benign or early malignant lesions, splenectomy is not principally indicated with distal pancreatectomy. Spleen preservation can be done either with (Warshaw 1988) or without splenic vessel resection (Kimura 1996).[25] Both techniques have been performed minimally invasively. The existing evidence shows that the vessel-sparing technique seems to be advantageous in reducing spleen-related complications.[25,26] There are no data about the rate of conversion from "intended" vessel preservation to vessel resection with or without splenectomy for technical reasons.

The main complication after both open and minimally invasive distal pancreatectomy (MIDP) is a postoperative pancreatic fistula (POPF). The rate of clinically significant POPF in large observational studies seems to be comparable,[5,6] whereas the best evidence from two randomized controlled trials (RCTs) has shown a trend to a higher fistula rate after MIDP of 36 versus 28% after ODP.[9] As with open distal pancreatectomy (DP), no evidence-based recommendations can be given regarding closure technique (stapler vs. non-stapler) or staple line reinforcement with glue or allogenic material.[15,27] Covering the resection margin with a ligamentum teres patch results in a reduced risk for severe POPF and reinterventions in ODP.[28] Yet, in our experience applying this technique in MIDP creates special technical difficulties, but this has not been investigated yet.

Conversion from minimally invasive to open surgery happens in about one of six cases and puts the patient at a higher risk of morbidity and mortality, particularly if conversion is due to emergency.[29,30] There have been several studies to find out pre- and intraoperative risk factors associated with a higher rate of conversion. A single-center retrospective analysis of 211 laparoscopic DPs identified, a preoperative diagnosis of malignant disease, surgeons LDPs experience (<15 cases) and associated resection of others organ, were independent risk factors for conversion, beside intraoperative findings like with adhesion, bleeding, vascular involvement and obesity.[31] In a large retrospective study, risk factors for conversion were found to be chronic pancreatitis, higher T stage tumors, higher BMI, lower serum albumin, and smoking habit.[29] The authors found significantly higher rates of overall complications for converted cases (55%) compared to MIDP (36%)

and ODP (44%) and a higher mortality of converted patients (2.2%) versus MIDP (0.3%, $p=0.006$) as well as versus ODP (0.9%, $p=0.16$). Another recently published study investigated outcomes after discrimination between elective and emergency conversion in a large international multicenter retrospective cohort.[30] While elective conversion happened in two-thirds with comparable short-term and oncological outcomes, emergency conversion was associated with a double overall morbidity (62 vs. 31%) and a trend to worse oncological outcome. In about 20% of converted cases, vascular resection was necessary. Although not all studies show a clear association between surgeons' experience and conversion rate, a training program can decrease the frequency of conversion significantly.[32,33]

Robotic technique for MIDP has been introduced since the beginning. A recent study has shown that robotic technique has been used in about one of four cases of MIDP in the USA in recent years.[3] Taken together, robotic DP seems to be at least as safe and feasible as laparoscopic DP with similar short- and long-term results.[34,35] There are data showing a reduced conversion rate and a positive impact on spleen and splenic vessel preservation of robotic compared to laparoscopic DP. A consensus of experts has used that for a strong recommendation in favor of RDP, spleen preservation is intended, despite a low level of evidence.[34]

Following an international meeting in Miami 2019, evidence-based guidelines on minimally invasive pancreatic resections have recently been published **(Table 1)**.[15] Although aiming to cover the subject comprehensively, the strength of recommendation remains low for most points addressed due to the limited evidence.

OWN RESULTS AND CONCLUSION

From 2009 until the end of 2020, we performed 201 minimally invasive distal pancreatectomies, 114 (57%) by conventional laparoscopy and 87 (43%) using a robot. Indications were benign cystic neoplasms in 25%, intraductal papillary mucinous neoplasm (IPMN) 17%, pancreatic neuroendocrine tumors (pNETs) 28%, pancreatic ductal adenocarcinoma (PDAC) 12%, chronic pancreatitis 8%, and various 10%. 18 (9%) were converted to open surgery. Overall morbidity was 42%. 11 (6%) patients underwent reoperation. A pancreatic fistula grade B and C developed in 23 patients (13%). There was no mortality.

Currently, a randomized controlled trial comparing MIDP and ODP for any indication is recruiting in our center to further increase the available evidence and more specifically define patients and indications suitable for MIDP.[36]

In our opinion, MIDP is a standard procedure with proven safety and feasibility, comparable morbidity and mortality, and oncologic equivalence to open surgery under certain conditions. No evidence exists to clearly determine

TABLE 1: The Miami International Evidence-Based Guidelines (2019) on minimal invasive distal and central pancreatectomy.

1a	MIDP for benign and low-grade malignant tumors is to be considered over ODP since it is associated with a shorter hospital stay, reduced blood loss, and equivalent complication rates.	1B
1b	Prospective data about the cost-effectiveness of MIDP compared to ODP is limited and requires further studies.	2C
1c	MIDP is associated with a better postoperative quality of life than ODP.	2B
2	MIDP for pancreatic ductal adenocarcinoma appears to be a feasible, safe, and oncologically efficient technique in experienced hands, although prospective comparative studies are lacking.	2B
3	There is no evidence regarding the use of vascular resection in MIDP. To address this question, data on patients' treatment and outcomes need to be entered in prospective registries and databases.	Expert opinion
4a	Both stapler and nonstapler closure can be used in MIDP as outcomes are comparable.	2C
4b	Evidence to support routine staple line reinforcement with any method or material is lacking.	2C
5	No studies exist specifically comparing minimally invasive spleen-preserving distal pancreatectomy with open spleen-preserving distal pancreatectomy.	2C
6	Both laparoscopic and robotic distal pancreatectomy are safe and feasible options. The use of either technique should be based on surgeons' experience and local resources.	2B

Summary of graded recommendations (1 = strong, 2 = weak recommendation, A = high, B = moderate, C = low quality of evidence).[15]

the appropriate timing or indication for conversion in MIDP. Elective conversion should be considered based on surgeon experience, concern for patient safety, or failure to progress. The surgeon is expected to have expertise in various methods to control bleeding in the event of hemorrhage that may require urgent conversion under certain conditions. It must be of concern that there is a substantial proportion of cases who undergo conversion to open surgery and have a worse outcome particularly if conversion is due to intraoperative complications. Therefore, particularly "emergency" conversion should be avoided best possible. Even though it is difficult to define strict selection criteria, there is no doubt that preoperatively known factors regarding the patient and the disease as well as surgeon's experience play a role for conversion. Accordingly, these factors should be meticulously taken into account for allocation of an individual case to a minimally invasive or open operation. But it may be more important to realize that for patients' sake, conversion to open surgery is not a "defeat" of the surgeon but a reasonable "exit strategy" to be performed soon and readily in an "elective" manner before complications force to do it as "emergency." This in mind, MIDP can today certainly be the procedure of choice for many cases.

REFERENCES

1. Cuschieri SA, Jakimowicz JJ. Laparoscopic pancreatic resections. Semin Laparosc Surg. 1998;5(3):168-79.
2. Merchant NB, Parikh AA, Kooby DA. Should all distal pancreatectomies be performed laparoscopically? Adv Surg. 2009;43:283-300.
3. Ellis RJ, Zhang LM, Ko CY, Cohen ME, Bentrem DJ, Bilimoria KY, et al. Variation in hospital utilization of minimally invasive distal pancreatectomy for localized pancreatic neoplasms. J Gastrointest Surg. 2020;24(12):2780-8.
4. Mehrabi A, Hafezi M, Arvin J, Esmaeilzadeh M, Garoussi C, Emami G, et al. A systematic review and meta-analysis of laparoscopic versus open distal pancreatectomy for benign and malignant lesions of the pancreas: it's time to randomize. Surgery. 2015 Jan;157(1):45-55.
5. Riviere D, Gurusamy KS, Kooby DA, Vollmer CM, Besselink MGH, Davidson BR, et al. Laparoscopic versus open distal pancreatectomy for pancreatic cancer. Cochrane Database Syst Rev. 2016;4(4):CD011391.
6. Røsok BI, de Rooij T, van Hilst J, Diener MK, Allen PJ, Vollmer CM, et al. Minimally invasive distal pancreatectomy. HPB (Oxford). 2017;19(3):205-14.
7. de Rooij T, van Hilst J, van Santvoort H, Boerma D, van den Boezem P, Daams F, et al. Minimally Invasive Versus Open Distal Pancreatectomy (LEOPARD): a multicenter patient-blinded randomized controlled trial. Ann Surg. 2019;269(1):2-9.
8. Björnsson B, Larsson AL, Hjalmarsson C, Gasslander T, Sandström P. Comparison of the duration of hospital stay after laparoscopic or open distal pancreatectomy: randomized controlled trial. Br J Surg. 2020;107(10):1281-8.
9. Korrel M, Vissers FL, van Hilst J, de Rooij T, Dijkgraaf MG, Festen S, et al. Minimally invasive versus open distal pancreatectomy: an individual patient data meta-analysis of two randomized controlled trials. HPB (Oxford). 2021;23(3):323-30.
10. Klompmaker S, de Rooij T, Koerkamp BG, et al. International validation of reduced major morbidity after minimally invasive distal pancreatectomy compared with open pancreatectomy. Ann Surg. 2021;274(6):e966-73.
11. Klompmaker S, van Zoggel DM, Watkins AA, Eskander MF, Tseng JF, Besselink MG, et al. Nationwide Evaluation of Patient Selection for Minimally Invasive Distal Pancreatectomy Using American College of Surgeons' National Quality Improvement Program. Ann Surg. 2017;266(6):1055-61.
12. Klompmaker S, Peters NA, van Hilst J, Bassi C, Boggi U, Busch OR, et al. Outcomes and risk score for distal pancreatectomy with celiac axis resection (DP-CAR): an International Multicenter Analysis. Ann Surg Oncol. 2019;26(3):772-81.
13. Bhat AS, Farrugia A, Marangoni G, Ahmad J. Multivisceral robotic resection: a glimpse into the future of minimally invasive abdominal surgery. BMJ Case Rep. 2020;13(8):e234887.
14. Sahakyan MA, Tholfsen T, Kleive D, Yaqub S, Kazaryan AM, Buanes T, et al. Laparoscopic distal pancreatectomy following prior upper abdominal surgery (pancreatectomy and prior surgery). J Gastrointest Surg. 2021;25(7):1787-94.

15. Asbun HJ, Moekotte AL, Vissers FL, Kunzler F, Cipriani F, Alseidi A, et al. The Miami International Evidence-based Guidelines on Minimally Invasive Pancreas Resection. Ann Surg. 2020;271(1):1-14.
16. van Hilst J, de Rooij T, Klompmaker S, Rawashdeh M, Aleotti F, Al-Sarireh B, et al. Minimally invasive versus open distal pancreatectomy for ductal adenocarcinoma (DIPLOMA): a Pan-European Propensity Score Matched Study. Ann Surg. 2019;269(1):10-7.
17. Sham JG, Gage MM, He J. Minimally invasive versus open distal pancreatectomy for ductal adenocarcinoma (DIPLOMA)-a difficult question to answer. Laparosc Surg. 2018;2:2.
18. van Hilst J, Korrel M, de Rooij T, Lof S, Busch OR, Koerkamp BG, et al. Oncologic outcomes of minimally invasive versus open distal pancreatectomy for pancreatic ductal adenocarcinoma: a systematic review and meta- analysis. Eur J Surg Oncol. 2019;45(5):719-27.
19. Zhang XF, Lopez-Aguiar AG, Poultsides G, Makris E, Rocha F, Kanji Z, et al. Minimally invasive versus open distal pancreatectomy for pancreatic neuroendocrine tumors: an analysis from the U.S. neuroendocrine tumor study group. J Surg Oncol. 2019;120(2):231-40.
20. de Rooij T, Sitarz R, Busch OR, Besselink MG, Hilal MA. Technical aspects of laparoscopic distal pancreatectomy for benign and malignant disease: Review of the literature. Gastroenterol Res Pract. 2015;2015:472906.
21. Asbun HJ, Van Hilst J, Tsamalaidze L, Kawaguchi Y, Sanford D, Pereira L, et al. Technique and audited outcomes of laparoscopic distal pancreatectomy combining the clockwise approach, progressive stepwise compression technique, and staple line reinforcement. Surg Endosc. 2020;34(1):231-9.
22. Cao F, Li J, Li A, Li F. Radical antegrade modular pancreatosplenectomy versus standard procedure in the treatment of left-sided pancreatic cancer: a systemic review and meta-analysis. BMC Surg. 2017;17(1):67.
23. Lee SH, Kang CM, Hwang HK, Choi SH, Lee WJ, Chi HS. Minimally invasive RAMPS in well-selected left-sided pancreatic cancer within Yonsei criteria: long-term (>median 3 years) oncologic outcomes. Surg Endosc. 2014;28(10):2848-55.
24. Sahakyan MA, Kleive D, Kazaryan AM, Aghayan DL, Ignjatovic D, Labori KJ, et al. Extended laparoscopic distal pancreatectomy for adenocarcinoma in the body and tail of the pancreas: a single-center experience. Langenbecks Arch Surg. 2018;403(8):941-8.
25. Nakata K, Shikata S, Ohtsuka T, Ukai T, Miyasaka Y, Mori Y, et al. Minimally invasive preservation versus splenectomy during distal pancreatectomy: a systematic review and meta-analysis. J Hepatobiliary Pancreat Sci. 2018;25(11):476-88.
26. Lee LS, Hwang HK, Kang CM, Lee WLJ. Minimally invasive approach for spleen-preserving distal pancreatectomy: a comparative analysis of postoperative complication between splenic vessel conserving and Warshaw technique. J Gastrointest Surg. 2016;20(8):1464-70.
27. Diener MK, Seiler CM, Rossion I, Kleeff J, Glanemann M, Butturini G, et al. Efficacy of stapler versus hand-sewn closure after distal pancreatectomy (DISPACT): a randomised, controlled multicentre trial. Lancet. 2011;377(9776):1514-22.
28. Hassenpflug M, Hinz U, Strobel O, Volpert J, Knebel P, Diener MK, et al. Teres ligament patch reduces relevant morbidity after distal pancreatectomy (the DISCOVER Randomized Controlled Trial). Ann Surg. 2016;264(5):723-30.

29. Nassour I, Wang SC, Porembka MR, Augustine MM, Yopp AC, Mansour JC, et al. Conversion of minimally invasive distal pancreatectomy: predictors and outcomes. Ann Surg Oncol. 2017;24(12):3725-31.
30. Lof S, Korrel M, van Hilst J, Moekotte AL, Bassi C, Butturini G, et al. Outcomes of elective and emergency conversion in minimally invasive distal pancreatectomy for pancreatic ductal adenocarcinoma: an International Multicenter Propensity Score-matched Study. Ann Surg. 2021;274(6):e1001-7.
31. Hua Y, Javed AA, Burkhart RA, Makary MA, Weiss MJ, Wolfgang CL et al. Preoperative risk factors for conversion and learning curve of minimally invasive distal pancreatectomy. Surgery. 2017;162(5):1040-7.
32. Balduzzi A, van der Heijde N, Alseidi A, Dokmak S, Kendrick ML, Polanco PM, et al. Risk factors and outcomes of conversion in minimally invasive distal pancreatectomy: a systematic review. Langenbecks Arch Surg. 2021;406(3):597-605.
33. de Rooij T, van Hilst J, Boerma D, Bonsing BA, Daams F, van Dam RM, et al. Impact of a nationwide training program in minimally invasive distal pancreatectomy (LAELAPS). Ann Surg. 2016;264(5):754-62.
34. Liu R, Wakabayashi G, Palanivelu C, Tsung A, Yang K, Goh BKP, et al. International consensus statement on robotic pancreatic surgery. Hepatobiliary Surg Nutr. 2019;8(4):345-60.
35. Alfieri S, Boggi U, Butturini G, Pietrabissa A, Morelli L, Di Sebastiano P, et al. Full robotic distal pancreatectomy: safety and feasibility analysis of a multicenter cohort of 236 patients. Surg Innov. 2020;27(1):11-8.
36. Department of General, Visceral and Transplantation Surgery University Hospital. [online] Available from: https://www.drks.de/drks_web/navigate.do?navigationId=trial.HTML&TRIAL_ID=DRKS00014011. [Last accessed November, 2021].

CHAPTER
12

Minimally Invasive Approach to Chronic Pancreatitis

Shreeyash Modak, GV Rao

■ INTRODUCTION

Open surgical approach is often used in operative management of chronic pancreatitis as it requires meticulous dissection and technically demanding reconstruction. Since its inception in 1980s, laparoscopy is being used more frequently for complex surgical procedures. The first laparoscopic pancreaticoduodenectomy was performed by Gagner and Pomp in 1994 for chronic pancreatitis.[1] Cuschieri et al. showed superiority of laparoscopy in distal pancreatosplenectomy in terms of shorter postoperative hospital stay and no increase in complications.[2] Since then, laparoscopic pancreatic surgeries are being performed in increasing numbers in high-volume centers with equivalent mortality and morbidity. Addition of robotics in the array of minimally invasive techniques has added advantages viz. three-dimensional vision, reduced operative fatigue, stabilization of tremors, and better ergonomics. Although the data on minimally invasive surgeries for chronic pancreatitis per se is limited, information from minimally invasive pancreatic surgeries overall can give us insight into its applicability. Surgery for chronic pancreatitis can be broadly categorized in (1) drainage procedures and (2) resectional procedures. In this chapter, we will discuss the role of minimally invasive surgery (MIS) in each of these procedures.

Major hurdles in an MIS procedure for chronic pancreatitis are as follows:
- *Exposure of pancreas*: Due to inflammatory nature of the disease, exposure of pancreas can be troublesome. It may lead to bleeding and injury to surrounding structure due to obscure anatomy. Absence of haptic feedback in MIS adds to the difficulty. Hence, in cases with recurrent attacks of acute pancreatitis and imaging showing ongoing inflammation, it would be prudent to choose open surgery over MIS.
- *Identification of pancreatic duct*: In open surgery, dilated pancreatic duct can be easily identified by palpating a depression in a relatively atrophic parenchyma. The same thing may not be possible in MIS and one must resort to either aspiration (which might lead to bleeding due to poor control in needle insertion) or intraoperative ultrasound (IOUS).
- *Hemostasis*: In open surgery after duodenal kocherization, surgeon can place his hand posterior to pancreatic head and by pressure alone achieve temporary hemostasis before definite control is done. This is important while doing head coring/resection, where pressure can be

applied with one hand and fine suturing or electrocoagulation with the other. This technique cannot be applied in MIS. The limited space to move instruments, unavailability of experienced assistant, obscuration of operative field, loss of pneumoperitoneum by continuous suction and decreased illumination due to pooled blood are some of the factors that can prompt open conversion.
- *Intracorporeal suturing*: To perform anastomosis and to achieve hemostasis one must be experienced in suturing techniques. Regular training in endotrainer can help in training the surgeon's hand which in turn helps to shorten the surgical time and decrease undue stress.

DRAINAGE PROCEDURES

Many drainage procedures have been described. Some of them are accompanied by partial resection/coring of pancreatic head. Ductal hypertension which is considered as a contributing factor for pain can be alleviated by such draining procedures, pancreatic duct stones can also be removed during the procedure. Few cases have associated chronic pseudocyst which also to be drained internally.

Minimally Invasive Lateral Pancreatojejunostomy (Partington-Rochelle)

This procedure is indicated in chronic pancreatitis without head mass, with stricture in head leading to a dilated duct. The duct is laid open along its entire length from head to tail and a side-to-side pancreatojejunostomy is done. The evidence for MIS lateral pancreatojejunostomy (LPJ) is largest among all drainage procedures. Reason for this is relatively less complexity involved in the surgery which can be adapted with a shorter learning curve. It was reported first by Kurian and Gagner, in a series of five laparoscopic lateral pancreatojejunostomy.[3] The two largest series from India are by Tantia et al. (17 cases) and Palanivelu et al. (12 cases). Tantia et al. reported 11.8% complication rate which included wound infection and internal hernia requiring surgery.[4] Palanivelu et al. did not report any major morbidity or mortality and nearly 85% patients had complete pain relief at a median follow-up of 4.4 years.[5] The same group reported a series of 39 cases in 2019 with satisfactory pain relief, operating time, and complication rate.[6] Khaled et al. also reported a small series of five patients with no mortality and 80% pain-free rate at 14 months follow-up.[7,8] As far as robotic surgery is concerned, only case reports are available.

Technique[5,6]

Patient is placed in reverse Trendelenburg's Lloyd-Davis position. A sandbag is placed under left side to give right lateral tilt. This optimizes the exposure. Ports are placed as shown in **Figure 1**.

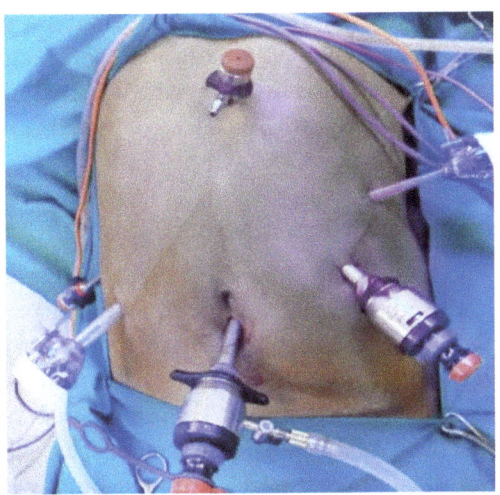

Fig. 1: Port position for laparoscopic drainage pictures.

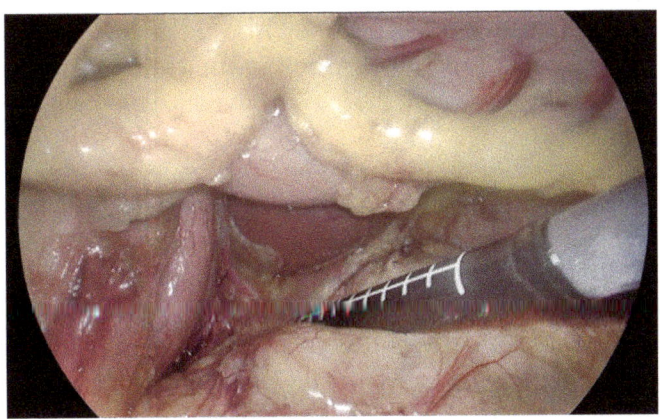

Fig. 2: Identification of duct by intraoperative pictures.

- *Exposure of pancreas*: The gastrocolic omentum is divided widely to expose pancreas from head to tail. All adhesions between posterior wall of stomach and pancreas are divided.
- *Identification and opening of pancreatic duct*: Pancreatic duct can be located by means of palpation with a blunt instrument, aspiration by lumbar puncture needle, or intraoperative ultrasound (IOUS) **(Fig. 2)**. Once located, duct is opened either with monopolar hook or ultrasonic sheers along its length. Stones are extracted with Maryland forceps.
- *Creation of Roux loop*: With an Endo GIA stapler Roux limb is created by transecting proximal jejunum at 20–25 cm distal to duodenojejunal (DJ) flexure. It is taken up in retrocolic fashion and aligned to pancreas with the blind end facing toward tail. Side-to-side jejunojejunostomy is done 50–60 cm distal to the blind end with Endo GIA stapler.

- *Pancreatojejunostomy*: Longitudinal jejunostomy is done according to the length of pancreatic duct. Side-to-side pancreatojejunostomy is performed in four layers. Outer first layer with interrupted 3-0 silk sutures. Inner second and third layers with 3-0 vicryl or prolene in running fashion followed by interrupted fourth layer with 3-0 silk.

Minimally Invasive Frey Procedure

Frey procedure is a hybrid procedure combining head resection/coring as well as drainage. It is indicated in inflammatory head mass associated with dilated duct. A minimum 8 mm diameter of pancreatic duct is a prerequisite. In addition to the operative steps of LPJ, head coring is done to remove 1.5 g of parenchymal tissue, leaving behind 0.5 cm rim of pancreas to safeguard duodenum and bile duct. As the procedure requires parenchymal resection, a meticulous hemostasis is required. A bipolar energy source and fine sutures 4-0/5-0 prolene are recommended to control hemorrhage from small perforators in the parenchyma. It is advisable to transfix gastroduodenal artery (GDA) both superiorly and inferiorly. Also, the gastrocolic trunk, which traverses the pancreatic head, needs to be transfixed to expose the pancreatic head completely. Kocherization is necessary to get better vision of head and uncinate process.

Tan et al. reported a series of nine cases out of which seven were completed in laparoscopy, while two had to be converted due to inability to locate duct. One patient had postoperative hemorrhage.[9] Killburn et al. in a series of four patients reported one Clavien-Dindo 4a complication in the form of pancreatojejunostomy leak and hemorrhage which required reoperation.[10] Senthilnathan et al. showed near-complete pain relief and weight gain in 15 patients who underwent laparoscopic Frey procedure. The average operating time and blood loss were 271 minutes and 290 mL, respectively. One patient had postoperative hemorrhage and two patients had pancreatic fistula.[6]

Minimally Invasive Beger Procedure/Berne Modification

Beger procedure or Berne modification is indicated for inflammatory head mass without dilatation of pancreatic duct.[11] The principle is to resect pancreatic head and uncinate process up to posterior pancreatic capsule and leave thin rim of tissue along medial border of duodenum. This also relieves biliary obstruction by exposing intrapancreatic portion of bile duct which can be included in the anastomosis if opened. The remnant pancreas is anastomosed to the jejunum in end-to-side fashion in Beger procedure, while in Berne's modification, the jejunum is anastomosed to the cored-out cavity which drains both pancreatic duct and bile duct. These procedures are more difficult to perform than Frey procedure due to increased complexity and dissection close to vital structures like bile duct and portomesenteric axis.

Available data regarding MIS Beger/Berne is limited. Khaled et al. has described one case with no postoperative morbidity and mortality.[7] Recently Cai et al. described a series of five laparoscopic Beger procedure done for chronic pancreatitis with inflammatory head mass. Median operative time was 275 minutes and average blood loss was 200 mL. One patient had grade B postoperative pancreatic fistula and one required reoperation for jejunojejunostomy bleeding.[12]

RESECTIONAL PROCEDURES

Pancreatoduodenectomy

Even though the first laparoscopic pancreaticoduodenectomy was done for chronic pancreatitis, the overall reported cases are less. Two main reasons for this are: (1) Indications for pancreaticoduodenectomy in chronic pancreatitis are limited and (2) in indicated cases, due to local inflammation and complexity of surgery, open approach is preferred over laparoscopic. From large studies all around the world, it has been shown that MIS pancreaticoduodenectomy is safe and feasible with complication rate comparable to open surgery. Laparoscopy can aid as a staging investigation in cases with chronic pancreatitis and a suspected malignancy in head of the pancreas, as there is a chance of inoperability in such patient.

Distal Pancreatectomy

Indication for distal pancreatectomy is focal pancreatitis limited to body and tail. This is usually associated with stricture in body region and neck. Spleen may or may not be preserved depending on degree of inflammation and technical difficulty in splenic vessel dissection. Due to the magnified vision, there is greater chance of splenic vessel preservation in laparoscopy then in open surgery. MIS distal pancreatectomy is routinely done for benign and premalignant lesions of pancreas and can be done even in chronic pancreatitis **(Figs. 3A and B)**.

Total Pancreatectomy with Islet Cell Autotransplantation

Primary indication for minimally invasive total pancreatectomy with islet cell autotransplantation is refractory pain of chronic pancreatitis with failed medical, endoscopic, and prior surgical procedure. It is a rarely done procedure due to associated severe morbidity in the form of labile diabetes. Zureikat et al. and Galvani et al. have reported three and six cases of MIS total pancreatectomy with or without islet cell transplantation, respectively.[13,14] They showed comparable perioperative outcomes. The techniques of resectional procedures are similar to those done for other indications.

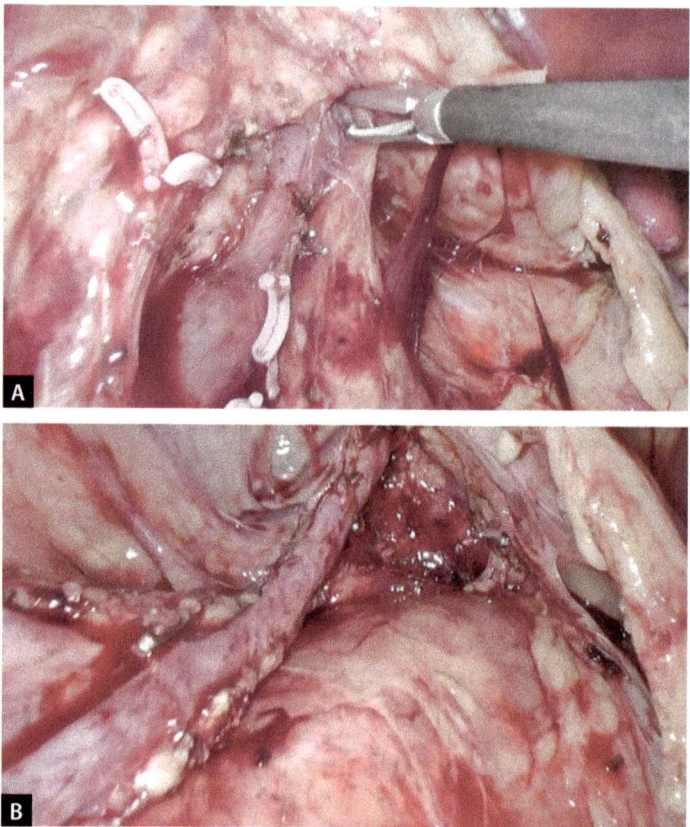

Figs. 3A and B: Distal pancreatectomy in chronic pancreatitis. Dense inflammation around the pancreas and completely bared splenic vein at the end of the procedure.

CONCLUSION

As the literature and evidence supporting MIS in chronic pancreatitis is limited and application of the same in clinical practice is not a routine practice, one must be cautious in the early stages of career. Sufficient experience in minimally invasive advanced gastrointestinal surgeries and open pancreatic surgeries is desirable. Selection of cases is of paramount importance. Distal pancreatectomy and lateral pancreatojejunostomy are the types of surgeries which require less complex parenchymal dissection and should be attempted in the early stages. As the experience of the surgical team increases, more complex cases requiring coring, head resection can be performed. One must be skilled in endoscopic suturing and familiar with different hemostatic techniques. Cross-sectional image reading must be learned to see peripancreatic inflammation, associated complications, and predict intraoperative difficulty. Last but not the least a good HD/4K camera system with good light source is preferable.

REFERENCES

1. Gagner M, Pomp A. Laparoscopic pylorus-preserving pancreatoduodenectomy. Surg Endosc. 1994;8(5):408-10.
2. Cuschieri A, Jakimowicz JJ, van Spreeuwel J. Laparoscopic distal 70% pancreatectomy and splenectomy for chronic pancreatitis. Ann Surg. 1996;223(3):280-5.
3. Kurian MS, Gagner M. Laparoscopic side-to-side pancreaticojejunostomy (Partington-Rochelle) for chronic pancreatitis. J Hepatobiliary Pancreat Surg. 1999;6(4):382-6.
4. Tantia O, Jindal MK, Khanna S, Sen B. Laparoscopic lateral pancreaticojejunostomy: our experience of 17 cases. Surg Endosc. 2004;18(7):1054-7.
5. Palanivelu C, Shetty R, Jani K, Rajan PS, Sendhilkumar K, Parthasarthi R, et al. Laparoscopic lateral pancreaticojejunostomy: a new remedy for an old ailment. Surg Endosc. 2006;20(3):458-61.
6. Senthilnathan P, Subrahmaneswara Babu N, Vikram A, Sabnis SC, Srivatsan Gurumurthy S, Anand Vijai N, et al. Laparoscopic longitudinal pancreatojejunostomy and modified Frey's operation for chronic calcific pancreatitis. BJS Open. 2019;3(5):666-71.
7. Khaled YS, Ammori BJ. Laparoscopic lateral pancreaticojejunostomy and laparoscopic Berne modification of Beger procedure for the treatment of chronic pancreatitis: the first UK experience. Surg Laparosc Endosc Percutan Tech. 2014;24(5):e178-82.
8. Khaled YS, Ammori MB, Ammori BJ. Laparoscopic lateral pancreaticojejunostomy for chronic pancreatitis: a case report and review of the literature. Surg Laparosc Endosc Percutan Tech. 2011;21(1):e36-40.
9. Tan CL, Zhang H, Li KZ. Single center experience in selecting the laparoscopic Frey procedure for chronic pancreatitis. World J Gastroenterol. 2015;21(11):12644-52.
10. Kilburn DJ, Chiow AKH, Leung U, Siriwardhane M, Cavallucci DJ, Bryant R, et al. Early experience with laparoscopic frey procedure for chronic pancreatitis: a case series and review of literature. J Gastrointest Surg. 2016;21(5):904-9.
11. Beger HG, Matsuno S, Cameron JL. Diseases of Pancreas – Current Surgical Therapy, 2nd edition. New York: Springer; 2016. pp. 391, 402, 404.
12. Cai H, Cai Y, Wang X, Peng B. Laparoscopic Beger procedure for the treatment of chronic pancreatitis: a single-centre first experience. BMC Surg. 2020;20(1):84.
13. Zureikat AH, Nguyen T, Boone BA, Wijkstrom M, Hogg ME, Humar A, et al. Robotic total pancreatectomy with or without autologous islet cell transplantation: replication of an open technique through a minimal access approach. Surg Endosc. 2015;29(1):176-83.
14. Galvani CA, Rodriguez Rilo H, Samamé J, Porubsky M, Rana A, Gruessner RW. Fully robotic-assisted technique for total pancreatectomy with an autologous islet transplant in chronic pancreatitis patients: results of a first series. J Am Coll Surg. 2014;218(3):e73-8.

Index

Page numbers followed by *f* refer to figure.

A

Abdomen 18
   lower 7, 35
Abdominal incision 99
Abdominal procedures, repeated 43
Abdominal surgery, major 1
Achilles' heel 6
Adenocarcinoma 23, 58
Adherent coagulated tissue 9*f*
Advanced bipolar vessel sealing
      device 14
Adventitia 92
Albumin 20
Anesthesia, choice of 1
Antecolic duodenojejunostomy,
      end-to-side 98
Appreciate arterial fluorescence 22
Ascites 80
Atrophic parenchyma 115

B

Balanced crystalloid 4
Basic surgical techniques 6
Berne's modification 118
Bile duct
   proliferation 25
   resection, indication for 51
Bile spillage 53
Biliary anatomy 27
Biliary ducts 26
Biliary tree mapping 26
Bilioenteric anastomosis 58
Bipolar coagulation 9, 10, 10*f*
Bipolar diathermy 7
Bipolar forceps 9*f*
   removal of 8
   replacement of 8
Bleeding control
   intraoperative 6
   techniques for 7
Bleeding, severe 9
Blood loss 6
   increased 8
Body mass index 105
Borderline resectable disease 78

C

Cadaver training 17
Cancerous tissues 24
Caudate lobe-first approach 34*f*
Cause, tumor dissemination 50
Celiac axis 108
Cells, malignant 26
Central hepatectomy 37
Central venous pressure 2, 3*f*
Chemotherapy, preoperative 25
Cholangiocarcinoma 24, 26
Cholangiography, intraoperative 28
Cholecystectomy 51
Chronic inflammation 66
Chronic pancreatitis 57, 115, 116,
      119, 120*f*
Cirrhosis 25
Clinical care pathways 60
Coagulation 2
Coagulogram 4
Colorectal liver metastases 37, 38, 40
   posterosuperior 42
   robotic resections for 44
   treatment of 37
Common bile duct 27, 70, 69*f*, 80
   lower 66
Common hepatic artery 69*f*, 88, 88*f*
Conventional laparoscopic
      instruments 57
Conventional radiology 60
Current laparoscopic surgery 15

D

Distal pancreatectomy 57, 105,
      119, 120*f*
Distal pancreatosplenectomy 115
Drainage procedures 116
Duct
   identification of 117*f*
   layer, anterior 97*f*
Duct-pancreatic suture, anterior 93
Duodenum 67
   first part of 83
   mobilization of 87*f*
   transection of 87*f*

Index

E

Emergency 112
Endoscopic ultrasound 80
Energy device 81
Epidural catheter removal 1
Extrahepatic ducts 27
Extremely precise dissection 79

F

Fibrillar oxidized cellulose 10
    placement of 10
Fibrosis 53
Fluorescence 22
    imaging
        basic principles in 20
        clinical applications of 20, 21
Fluorescence
    guided surgery 20
    type of 23
Fluorescent regions, identification of 25
Fluorophore 21
    administration 22
    dye 20
Fourth robotic port 53
Frey procedure 118

G

Gallbladder 68, 69f
    cancer 50
        managing 50
        robotic surgery in 53
        surgery of 54
Gastric artery clipped and divided, right 86f
Gastrocolic ligament 83, 106
    division of 84f
Gastrocolic momentum 67
Gastrocolic trunk insertion 85f
Gastroduodenal artery 69f, 70f, 83, 90f, 118
    junction of 88f
Gastroenterostomy 58
Gastroepiploic artery, right 84
Gastroepiploic vein, right 83
Gastrointestinal surgeries 16
Gastrojejunostomy 65, 68, 98
Glissonean branches 32
Glissonean pedicles 34
    anterior 35f
    division of 35f
    posterior 35f
Glissonean
    tree 32
    trunk 34, 34f

H

Hand-assisted system 11, 12
Healthcare system 60
Healthy liver 39
Hemihepatectomy 32
    completion of right 36f
Hemorrhage, postoperative 118
Hemostasis 18, 108, 115
    bipolar for 41f
Hemostatic devices 12
Hemostatic stay sutures 89
Hepatectomy
    laparoscopic right 32
    major 38
Hepatic artery, right 68, 69f
Hepatic hilum 32, 34, 35f
Hepatic inflow, total 4
Hepatic liver dysfunction 2
Hepatic segments
    boundaries of 26
    identification of 26
Hepatic tumors 25
Hepatic vein 10, 32
    middle 34, 35f
Hepaticojejunostomy 65, 68, 96, 99f
Hepatobiliary surgery 22
    clinical applications in 23
Hepatocellular carcinoma 6, 23
Hepatocytes, compressed 24
Hepatoduodenal ligament 18, 51, 53
    lymphatic clearance of 52f
Hyper eye medical system 23
Hypochondrium 32
    left 33f

I

Incidentally diagnosed gallbladder 52
Incisionless cholangiography 27f
Indocyanine green 16, 20, 21
    fluorophore administration 21
    role of 20
    systems 22
Inflammatory adhesions 53
Inflammatory nature 115
Inflow occlusion technique 8
Infracolic compartment 67
Initiating robotic pancreaticoduodenectomy 78
Instantaneous bipolar coagulation 10
Intensive care unit 72
Intra-abdominal pressure 8, 11
    increase of 8
    low 8
Intracorporeal suturing 116

Index

Intraductal papillary mucinous neoplasm 66, 110
Intrahepatic biliary anatomy 28*f*
Intraoperative bleeding 14
Intravascular volume, management of 40
Intravenous fluid 4
Ischemia reperfusion injury 2
Islet cell autotransplantation 119

J

Jaundice 66
Jejunal stay suture 95
Jejunal vein, first 68
Jejunojejunostomy 68
   fashioned 68
   side-to-side 117

K

Kidney injury, acute 1
Kocher maneuver 85

L

Laparoscopic bile duct 52
Laparoscopic bleeding control 11
Laparoscopic caudodorsal magnified view 33
Laparoscopic clarity ultrasonic surgical aspirator system 14
Laparoscopic distal
   pancreatectomy 106
   pancreatosplenectomy, operative technique for 106
Laparoscopic drainage pictures, port position for 117*f*
Laparoscopic extended
   cholecystectomy 51
   major hepatectomy 42
Laparoscopic hepatectomy 6, 11, 14, 15, 17, 18
   initiating 14
Laparoscopic instruments 108
Laparoscopic left lateral sectionectomy 39*f*
Laparoscopic liver
   resection 1-3, 6, 15, 16, 37, 42
   surgery 6, 20
Laparoscopic major hepatectomies 40
Laparoscopic minor liver resections 38
Laparoscopic pancreatic resection 65
Laparoscopic pancreaticoduodenectomy 65, 79, 84*f*-86*f*, 88*f*, 90*f*, 95*f*-98*f*, 100
   first 115

   indications 66
   uncinate dissection 92*f*
Laparoscopic pancreatoduodenectomy 65, 73
Laparoscopic parenchymal sparing 40
Laparoscopic procedure 54, 68
Laparoscopic reoperation 53
Laparoscopic resection 42, 58
Laparoscopic surgery 50, 59
   concerns of 16
Laparoscopic techniques, application of 73
Laparoscopic ultrasonic sears 14
Laparoscopic ultrasound 18
Laparoscopy, staging 60
Laparotomy 66
   decreases 11
Lesions, malignant 58, 109
Ligamentum teres 69*f*, 108
Lipoprotein 20
Liver 10*f*, 80
   enzymes, monitoring of 4
   function 1
   injury, chemotherapy-induced 43
   lesions 25
   malignancies, secondary 23
   mobilization 40
   parenchyma 7, 9, 12, 22, 32, 34
   resection 2, 15, 17, 17, 24, 51, 53*f*
      laparoscopic repeated 43
      open 38
      partial 37
      treatment option for 44
   segment
      negative staining technique for 27*f*
      visualization 26
   surgery 25
   transection 28
   tumor
      identification 23
      localization 23
Lobe, right 35
Local inflammation 119
Low central venous pressure, challenges of 3
Low-grade malignancies 66
Low-voltage electrical cautery 32
Lung 80

M

Malign tumors 105
Malignant disease, diagnosis of 109
Maryland bipolar forceps 81
Maryland forceps 117
Mesopancreas 100
Metastatic liver tumors 24, 25

Index

Meticulous hemostasis 66, 118
Miami international evidence-based guidelines 111
Mid-bile duct cancer 66
Minimal access surgery, advantages of 65
Minimally invasive
   distal pancreatectomy 105, 109
   frey procedure 118
   lateral pancreatojejunostomy 116
   liver resections 44
   pancreatic surgery 58, 59, 61
      changing trends in 57
      evidence-based indications for 59
   pancreaticoduodenectomy 65, 78-80, 102
      evidence for 101
   procedures 37
   surgery 50, 58
      cost-effective 60
   techniques, application of 37
   treatment 37
Minimizing blood loss 7
Monopolar electrode with saline irrigation 11
Monopolar scissors, curved 81
Mucinous cystic neoplasms 66
Mucosa
   anastomosis 71f
   technique, duct to 68

N

Neoadjuvant chemotherapy 39
Non-anatomical segmental resection, laparoscopic marking for 52f

O

Oncological surgery 54
Ondocyanine green 20
Open distal pancreatectomy 105
Organic anion-transporting polypeptide 24
Organoscopy 57

P

Pancreas 89, 106, 107
   adenocarcinoma of 59
   exposure of 115, 117
   neck of 67
   preparation of 107f
   stapler division of 107f
   superior border of 88f
   uncinate process of 81

Pancreatectomy, total 119
Pancreatic bed 59
Pancreatic cancer 60
   staging of 60
Pancreatic diseases, diagnostic laparoscopy for 57
Pancreatic duct 93, 116, 118
   cannulation of 97f
   identification of 115
   opening of 117
   stenting of 94
Pancreatic fistula 78
   postoperative 78
Pancreatic head 118
Pancreatic neck 70f
   division of 89, 91f
   transected 70f
Pancreatic necrosis 59
   infected 61
Pancreatic parenchyma, anterior 93
Pancreatic stent 71f
Pancreatic surgeons 57, 61
Pancreatic surgery 57, 61
Pancreatic tumors, benign 59
Pancreaticoduodenal artery, inferior 93
Pancreaticoduodenal vein
   inferior 68
   superior 68
Pancreaticoduodenectomy 78, 119
   open 68, 101
Pancreaticojejunal anastomosis, completed 72f
Pancreaticojejunal duct 71f
Pancreaticojejunostomy 65, 68, 78
Pancreatitis, acute necrotizing 59
Pancreatoduodenectomy 57, 119
   popularization of 65
Pancreatojejunostomy 93, 118
   lateral 116
   side-to-side 116
Parenchyma 38, 118
   tissue 118
   transection 7, 40
Periampullary lesions 66
Peripheral portal pedicle, bleeding of 10
Periportal dissection 86
Periportal nodes, dissection of 89f
Peritoneum 80
Phlebostatic axis 3f
Photodynamic eye 23
Pneumoperitoneum 14, 32, 108
   loss of 116
   pressure 7
Polydioxanone 81
Porta hepatis 83

Portal lymphadenectomy 100
Portal vein
   dissection 70*f*
   injection 26
   left border of 88
   resection 41*f*
Positive end-expiratory pressure 3
Posterior duct
   layer 96*f*
   pancreatic suture 93
   suture 94*f*
Post-hepatectomy bile leak 28*f*
Posthepatectomy hepatic failure, risk of 18
Potentially curative surgery 25
Preferred suture materials 81
Pringle maneuver 19*f*, 32
Prograsp forceps 81
Pulmonary artery hypertension 3
Pylorus 98
Pylorus-preserving pancreaticoduodenectomy 82*f*, 83

R

Radical surgery, goals of 51
Recurrent colorectal metastases 43
Remnant liver 35*f*
Renal function 4
Renal vessels 108
Resectional procedures 119
Respiratory function, preservation of 1
Retropancreatic tunnel 67
Right portal vein for pedicle control, dissection of 41*f*
Robot-assisted distal pancreatectomy 79
Robotic approach 53
   disadvantages of 100
Robotic cholecystectomy 27
Robotic hepatobiliary surgery 26
Robotic liver
   resections 44
   surgery 38
Robotic pancreaticoduodenectomy 79, 84*f*-86*f*, 88*f*, 90*f*-92*f*, 95*f*-98*f*
   evidence for 101
   patient position for 81
   port position for 81
   surgical equipment for 81
Robotic port 81
   placement 82*f*
Robotic pylorus preserving pancreaticoduodenectomy
   operative procedure of 83
   setup for 82*f*

Robotic reconstruction 79
Robotic surgery, advent of 79
Roux loop, creation of 117

S

Safe laparoscopic hepatectomy 7
Segmentectomy, right posterior 41*f*
Specimen extraction 81
Splenectomy 109
Splenic artery 107
   division of 108*f*
Splenic vein, preparation of 107*f*
Stroke volume variation 3
Subcellular organelle 21
Subphrenic space, right 35
Suction catheter 10*f*
   tip 9*f*
Superior mesenteric
   artery 78
   vein 83, 85*f*, 91, 92
Supplementary technique 11
Suture hitching 69*f*

T

T metastatic disease 80
Technical competence, achievement of 61
Technical difficulty scoring system 15*f*
Transfusion rates 40
Trendelenburg's position 53
Trendelenburg's Lloyd-Davis position 116
Trocar placement 33*f*

U

Ultrasonic dissector 93
Uncinate dissection 71*f*, 90
   completion of 71*f*

V

Vascular stapler, use of 41*f*
Vena cava, inferior 3, 67
Viscoelastic coagulation 2
Vision, two-dimensional 79
Vitamin K 1

W

Water-soluble fluorophore 20
Winslow foramen 18
Wound infection 116

Y

Yonsei criteria 109

EU GSPR Authorised Reprsentative
Logos Europe, 9 rue Nicolas Poussin
1700, La Rochelle, France
Phone: +33 (0) 6 67 93 73 78
E-mail: contact@logoseurope.eu

www.ingramcontent.com/pod-product-compliance
Ingram Content Group UK Ltd.
Pitfield, Milton Keynes, MK11 3LW, UK
UKHW050428150426
5217IPUK00019B/1295